Enriched food combat Child Malnutrition

By

Manmeet Kaur

ACKNOWLEDGEMENT

First of all I bow down in complete submission before "Waheguruji" whose blessing hand on me enables me to achieve the seemingly unachievable goals.

I feel a deep sense of gratitude and obligation to my venerable supervisor Dr Tarvinder Jeet Kaur, Professor Department of Home Science K.U.K, for her luminous guidance, constant encouragement and sublime suggestions. Words are not enough to express what I owe her as she even spared her precious personal family time to help me out at every step of my research work.

I pay my most sincere regards to my respectable colleagues from Pt.ClS. Govt.P.G College Karnal, Dr Saroj Nain, Dr Mamta Bhardwaj, Dr Madhulikha, Dr Adarsh Panjeta, Dr Ritu Jaglan and Dr Balwan Singh for extending immeasurable help and scholarly guidance at every crucial step of the research work. A special thanks to Dr Neeraj Batish, Associate Professor Department of Law, K.U.K and Dr Sulochana Batish, Assistant Professor Department of History D.V.A College Karnal. Here, I would also like to take the opportunity to express my thanks to my friends whose jovial and cooperative attitude always kept me in a light mood during the work.

It is a matter of pleasure for me to thank Mr. Jagdish Singh Chief Consultant Pathologist and Microbiologist at Singh Sabha path lab and Mrs. Kirti Mongia (nursing sister) for their untiring support and precision in work that made the collection of blood samples smooth and absolute.

I would like to thank Mrs Rajni Pasricha Programme Officer ICDS and Mrs. Krishna Dalal, Supervisor ICDS, at Karnal district who introduced me to the local children who were the subjects for my study.

I express immense thanks to all teaching, non-teaching staff and research scholars of the department of Home science K.U.K, who overtly or covertly were instrumental in facilitating the completion of this work.

I would also like to record my thanks to Mr B.K Aneja, my statistician, for his excellent and dedicated services in connection with data analysis and Mr Ajay Gupta for his editing skills in sketching out the face of this study. The study would not have come to successful completion without their help.

Words fail in conveying my deep sense of gratitude to my husband Sardar Amrit Singh who has always been there to bear the burden of family responsibilities to ensure my long hours of concentration at my research work and held my hand to overcome every obstacle that could hinder my progress. Completion of this task would not have been possible without the love and support of my kids Gurasis kaur and Jeffraj Singh whose innocent smiles helped me smile in the hours of stressed intellectual labour.

My heartfelt gratitude cannot be captured in words for the love, affection and unflinching support and valuable advices of my chachu Sardar Charanjeet Singh ji. Words can never truly portray the constant encouragement and the support of my father-in-law Sardar Satwant Singh ji and mother-in-law Kuldeep Kaur ji.

There are certain people in everyone's life towards whom sense of deepest gratitude is beyond words. My gratefulness is towards my brother Harpreet Singh and sister Gurdiksha Kaur whose love and support made my journey least obstacle ridden. A special thanks to my Masi's Sardarni Surinder Kaur ji, Harbans Kaur ji and Kuldeep Kaur ji who used to be pillar of strength for me.

I shall be failing in my duty if I do not pay my gratitude towards all of my subjects and their parents who enthusiastically volunteered to be a part of this research work and remained consistent throughout intervention period. Hope my research work will contribute however small the fraction is, to the upliftment of such vulnerable sections of society at large and enable then to live a healthy life.

I would like to dedicate my work to my beloved parents, Sardar Inderjeet Singh Rikhi ji and late Sardarni Gurmail Kaur ji, as it was their dream and their words of inspiration and encouragement provided me with the strength, courage and patience required to realise this dream.

MANMEET KAUR

LIST OF TABLES

LIST OF FIGURES

LIST OF FLOW CHARTS

CONTENTS

Acknowledgement

List of Tables

List of Figures

List of Photos

List of flow chart

CHAPTER	DESCRIPTION	PAGE NO.

ABSTRACT

Two hundred undernourished pre-school children, purposively selected from Karnal district, stratified into five strata of forty units with twenty control and twenty experimental each constituted the basis of the study. Experimental trial sub-groups were named as per their nutrition intervention viz. Probiotic Supplemented Group (PSG), Value-added Food Supplemented Group (VAFSG), Nutrition Education (NE), Nutrition Education and Probiotic Supplemented Group (NE+PSG), Nutrition Education and Value-added Food Supplemented Group (NE+VAFSG). No nutrition intervention was given to the pre-school children of corresponding control sub-groups. A self-designed questionnaire was devised to obtain information regarding socio-economic status, food habits, clinical symptoms, anthropometric and bio-chemical parameters. Nutritional knowledge of the mothers of pre-schoolers was also assessed through self-designed questionnaire. Maximum (29.5%) children belonged to three years age group followed by four years (28%), five years (22%) and six years (20.5%).

Mean per cent intake of all the food groups (except pulses and sugar) and nutrients (except protein and iron in 3 years age group) was found to be inadequate before and after trial period as compared to RDA. Intervention trials showed significant change ($p \leq 0.01$ to $p \leq 0.05$) in the mean intake of all the food groups (except fats and oil) among 3 years age-group subjects at the end of intervention trial. While in experimental subjects of 4-6 years age-group, significant change ($p \leq 0.01$ to $p \leq 0.05$) in mean food intake was observed in all the food groups (except pulses, GLV and fruits) after the intervention trial period. At the end of intervention trials, all the nutrients (except fats and β-carotene) brought significant improvements ($p \leq 0.01$ to $p \leq 0.05$) in mean daily intake of nutrients among 3 years age-group. The acceptable level of supplementation varied in all the food preparations, *Dalia* was the best acceptable preparation at 1.7 per cent with spirulina supplementation, while acceptable level of *Poshtik bhel* and biscuits were at 16.6 per cent and 25 per cent with an incorporation of roasted soybean and soybean flour. Perusal of the data (Height) for the intervention with probiotics (PSG), value added foods (VAFSG) and nutrition education along with value-added foods (NE+VAFSG) have also shown comparatively good signs of significant change (p≤0.01) in the mid and end of the study period. Results revealed that significant improvement in weight was noticed among the experimental sub-groups of PSG, VAFSG, NE, NE+VAFSG at all stages of trial. Further, analysis of the data (BMI) confirmed, VAFSG most effective intervention treatment with 17.2 per cent improvement. Results of arm circumference showed maximum gain in mean per cent among the experiment sub-groups of PSG (11.7%) followed by NE+PSG (5.8%) and VAFSG (4.3%) after 120 days of experimental trial. Significant (p≤0.01) change was noticed in all the experimental trial groups except experimental sub-group of NE and control group of NE+VAFSG after completion of the trial. The data of subscapular skin fold thickness revealed that significant (p≤0.01) increment in VAFSG and NE+VAFSG experimental group at D/A and B/A stage of nutrition intervention. Triceps skin fold thickness observed values revealed that the mean per cent change was gradually improved in all the experimental groups (except NE+PSG). Whereas statistical analysis revealed that the values of experimental group of PSG (D/A and B/A), VAFSG (B/D, D/A and B/A) and NE+VAFSG (D/A) were significantly (p≤0.01) improved.

Biochemical parameters were collected to observe effects of various intervention trials on the bodies of pre-school children. Comparatively, mean per cent change (Total protein) was found to be the highest among NE + VAFSG (5.4%), followed by VAFSG (4.7%), NE + PSG (4.1%) and PSG (2.8%). Perusal of data further concluded that NE+VAFSG and VAFSG experimental sub-groups represented significant (p≤0.01) difference for B/D, D/A and B/A. For NE+PSG experimental group B/D and B/A have shown a good impact (p≤0.01).

The highest mean change (serum albumin) was observed for B/A (13.3%) in NE+PSG treatment group in the experimental sample followed by 12.3 per cent in B/A for experimental sample of NE+VAFSG and 6.9 per cent in B/A of VAFSG experimental subjects. NE+PSG has shown maximum (13.3%) efficacy of nutrition intervention in the estimation of serum albumin. The comparative analysis indicated maximum (9.3%) mean percentage change, noticed in serum globulin (at D/A), in case of experimental sub-group which had been intervened with nutrition education along with probiotic supplementation. Highest mean percentage change in haemoglobin of the order of 25.7 per cent was identified in the experimental sample of N.E+PSG.

Apart from this intervention sub-group, some others have also shown good impact i.e. 17.9 per cent by VAFSG, 13 per cent by N.E+ VAFSG and 11.1 per cent by PSG. As it is evident through highly significant values of t-static (p≤0.01) that NE+PSG and VAFSG have shown much greater impact as seen during the entire experiment period.

Statistical analysis revealed that highly significant (p≤0.01) improvement was noticed in mean knowledge, practice and attitude scores after imparting nutrition education to mothers of the respondents. Comparatively maximum improvement in KAP scores was found among NE+VAFSG followed by NE+PSG and NE

For weight-for-age, the data shows that there had been a sharp decrease (47%) in the cases of severe malnourishment after imparting nutrition interventions, which got shifted to moderate (25%) and normal (22%) categories. The data recorded for height-for-age revealed that 16, 16 and 68 per cent of the experimental subjects were in the category of normal, severely and moderately malnourished before imparting nutrition interventions, whereas the nominal increments (2% and 7%) were found in normal and moderate category after the completion of the experimental trial. The data for weight-for-height revealed that in the experimental group, 46 per cent moved to the normal category of weight-for-height, out of which 31 per cent were from moderate category and the rest were from severely malnourished category. Only 8 and 5 per cent of the respondents were in moderate and severe category after 120 days of experimental trial.

CHAPTER - 1
INTRODUCTION

Undernourishment is mainly due to the inability to receive high-quality food for consumption or when an individual is not getting the desired level of calories, protein, or micronutrients through various sources. The micronutrient deficiencies, stunting, wasting, and being underweight constitute the term 'Undernutrition' (WHO-2016). "Undernutrition is determined by low weight-for-age, low weight-for-height, and low height-for-age (WHO,2006)". Undernutrition has multidimensional aspects associated with deteriorated sensory-motor capacity, impaired cognitive functions, reproductive disorders, and social development issues with an overall decrease in quality of the life of individual. The undernutrition phenomenon escalates worldwide health confrontations linked to exceptional care, infirmity, and death.

Undernutrition is the main causative factor with a pessimistic impact on the child's growth, and it also impairs the school recital and efficiency of the child. More than 2 million children die due to malnutrition every year before they reach the age of five. The World Health Organization (WHO) has reported that out of 178 million malnourished children globally, about 20 million are severely malnourished affecting 3.5-5 million death annually among children less than 5years. Furthermore, Asia, particularly south-central Asia, accounts for 70% of the world's wasted infants (UNICEF-World Bank 2012).

Undernutrition in children less than five years in India is dominating globally and about double of Sub-Saharan Africa (World Bank-2014). 151 million children were stunted globally in 2017, with approximately 24% of children (less than five years) experiencing stunted growth in low & middle income countries (UNICEF, 2018). "The Global Nutrition Report (2018)" reiterates the emergency of undernutrition in the nation as India is on the top for stunted children.

Undernutrition is a focal communal health indicator and prospective source of high disease-prone or morality status in South Asia. Persuasive data suggests that malnutrition is the primary cause of underweight, wasting, and stunting, with tremendous growing consequences among society's vulnerable section. India has the maximum proportion of underweight children with 2-5 years of age.

1

It has also been reported that India recorded 25.5 million wasted children, along with Nigeria 3.4 million, and Indonesia, with 3.3 million children (Phungwayo, *et.al.*2021).Focus on the early stages of life is a matter of more significant concern as malnutrition affects the child's growth and overall development and the several indicators of child growth. Good nutrition for all is the requisite constituent to maintain good health. A healthy and economically viable diet providing optimal nutrition is the need of the hour for promoting salubrious life.

The World Bank UNICEF, and WHO divulge that the world is still far from being malnutrition free. The "Joint World Bank" issues a print in March 2019 presenting the markers of stunting and wasting amongst <5 years age group child and consistent progress has been observed in the target to achieve the "World Health Assembly goals set for 2025" and scaling up movement target plan for 2030 (UNICEF-World Bank-2019). Though undernutrition is apparent in varied ways, the direction and pathways to hinder are almost identical: varied nutritious and safe food at an early age, sufficient nutrition to the mother during and after pregnancy, healthy environment for the children with proper hygiene and sanitation all around. The development assessment evaluates children's health and nutritional status and provides significant measures to decide prospective action. However, other similarly significant malnutrition forms less evident to the naked eye-specifically, are deficiencies of vital vitamins and minerals. The risk of infection and contagious disease, and moderate undernutrition deteriorates each immune system segment.

Nutrition evolution in India was reconsidered by the "U.N.'s Food and Agriculture Organization" in 2006 with documented data for ongoing transition amongst society's wealthier segments (Kennedy G, 2017).To evaluate and assess the remaining nutrition and health hygiene challenges, India's government has launched the National Nutrition Mission (POSHAN ABHIYAN) in March 2018 (National Health Portal-India). The government has fulfilled its necessary obligations by forming determined goals and putting considerable efforts to introduce an effective financial plan for better nutrition that transforms into well-built immunity, illness-free, and superior health. In 2012, the WHA(World Health Assembly) approved an inclusive execution plan for the young infant, child, and maternal nutrition (lactating mother) that intensified six global targets related to priority nutrition levels to be attained by 2025

(WHO-2014). Worldwide major organizations, NGOs, local governments, and World Bank need to influence and take up the issues to ultimately eradicate malnutrition from the specified areas for the economic development of society and a healthy environment all over.

The child undernutrition problem is mainly concerned with middle and low-income countries, where one-third of the infants are expected to be malnourished. (Mohseni.*et.al* 2019).Child growth and development is globally recognized as critical in nutritional status and health in growing populations. Children's dietary needs are unique and demand special attention because of their rapid growth and development. Preschool children require persistent thought worldwide in this direction. This age group needs unique nutritional requirements for their growth and overall development. Reducing child malnutrition requires economically viable nutritious food. A major focus should be on addressing the dietary needs of particularly vulnerable groups and the simultaneous increase in the demand and availability of value-added food products to improve their health, growth, development, and maintain future health and efficiency. It is mandatory to move ahead with the exponential growth and use of particular food commodities or to formulate value-added food preparations for a malnourished preschool group of children. Therefore, the availability of nutritious value-added recipes developed mainly for preschool children is the need of the hour.

Value-added supplemented nutrition-sensitive food approaches are a must for improving the potential of the diet and eradication of malnutrition. Value-addition or supplemented recipes can enhance the nutritional value of the food by adding functional ingredients and improving their sensory attributes, which is the fundamental objective of value addition in the dietary system.

Spirulina is one of the blue-green microalgae which is indigenous to Africa and used worldwide nowadays. Spirulina genre can serve as an excellent substitute for various uses allied to nutritious food and therapeutic formulations of food which transform immune function and control numerous diseases (Karkos. *et.al*.2011). Spirulina is considered one of the most excellent protein sources in gram protein per cultivable land ratio (Siva Kiran *et al.*, 2015). As per NASA report 1kg of spirulina carries nutrition power equivalent to 1000 kg of vegetables and fruits. NASA and the

European space agency MELISSA recommended spirulina as a significant food and nutrition supplement. Spirulina can be used from infancy to adulthood for both genders, i.e., male and female. However, its effects mainly manifest in the young growing child, especially at the weaning and preschool stage. Spirulina is a vital complete food source of efficient nutrients with all every essential amino acids along with beta-carotene. 4 per cent decline in bitot's spot among 50,000 pre-school children was reported by Seshadari, 1993 on feeding one gram of dried spirulina for six to thirteen months. Value-added food product formulated with spirulina, cornflour, and wheat flour at 5,5 and 90 per cent concentration respectively was found to be well accepted and can safely be recommended (Vijayarani *et al.,*2012). The microalgae are supplemented in various food formulations. The blue-green micro-algae can be proposed to alleviate problems related to malnutrition and being rich in multiple nutrients, is simple to produce economically and can supplement many traditional foods (Hug & Weid 2011).

30 undernourished children (18-36 months of age) fed with 10 g spirulina daily, for nine months, resulted into better improvement in HAZ (Normal) (Masuda. *et al.* 2014). Féfé Khuabi Matondo *et al.* (2016) also observed significant growth for weight-for-height and weight-for-age along with significant improvement in total proteins, albumin, and corpuscular volume among the interventional group intervened with 10gm of spirulina daily.

Onubi *et al.* (2015) discussed the advantages of consuming prebiotics (produced by probiotics) in terms of weight and height gain, particularly in malnourished children in developing countries. Furthermore, the children's growth curves in the probiotic groups were considerably higher than others in the comparison group, implying that probiotics aid in the compensatory growth of children with stunting.

Soybean, a legume grown in subtropical, tropical, and moderate temperatures, is considered to have maximum protein content of all food crops and equal protein availability in animal feed. Biscuits are one of the oldest bakery products with cheaper worldwide demands, especially among children and other age groups and are ready to eat at any time. Wheat or *maida*, the main ingredient that constitutes most biscuits, lacks in essential amino acid lysine. In contrast, soybean is a better alternative, well-off in lysine and sulphur-containing amino acids. Supplementation of soybean in

4

biscuits or other forms of food is very common in most parts of the nations and especially suited for the economically weaker sections of society.

Supplementation or value–addition may not always be productive on its own. The intervention studies need to be accompanied by awareness through nutrition education, and it must propagate nutrient-rich food consumption, especially for the target population. In general parents do not possess enough nutritional knowledge regarding means for proper nutrition along with health-seeking and health care behaviours. Recommendation for a healthy diet in qualitative and quantitative terms and dissemination of good knowledge regarding the quantum and sizes of servings per day must be identified by each individual. It must be understood that the attribute characteristics rely on the natural intake utilization of the nutrients in the food, and quantitative indicators comprise the estimation of the quantity of nutrients necessary to consume.

Malnutrition among children less than five years is a foremost concern for health officials. There is a need to empower public health interventions for mild malnutrition cases and vulnerable populations along with forceful local implementation and evaluation of strategies. Hence, the critical status of undernourished children in the target group stresses, the significance of the value-added supplemented food formulations and nutrition education in improving the nutritional level of the undernourished children among the vulnerable group. In order to fill the gap in the existing knowledge the present research project is proposed for partial fulfilment of the research. Below stated are the proposed objectives of the present study.

1. To assess nutritional status of undernourished children.
2. To develop enriched food preparations and nutrition education material for nutrition intervention.
3. To intervene undernourished children with nutrition interventions.
4. To study the efficacy of nutrition interventions on nutritional status of undernourished children.

CHAPTER - 2
REVIEW OF LITERATURE

The following subheadings were used to organise the review of literature relevant to the current study:

2.1 Undernutrition: An Overview

2.2 Undernutrition in the World: A Global Scenario

2.3 Undernutrition: A National Scenario

2.4 Undernutrition: A Regional Scenario

2.5 Undernutrition in pre-school children

2.6 The role of probiotic in enhancing the nutritional status of undernourished children

2.7 Development and sensory evaluation of value-added food preparations

2.8 Role of feeding interventions in improving nutritional status of children

2.9 Impact of nutrition education and counselling

2.1 Undernutrition: An overview:

Nutrition is a vital column for one's growth and development. Undernutrition is primarily caused by a lack of dietary energy; irrespective of any additional specific nutrient is a limiting factor. Undernutrition is often replaced with the term malnutrition which means an impairment of health, either because of deficit or excess, or by an imbalance of nutrients.

Measures of child malnutrition are used to track the development and progress of children. Analysis of child malnutrition during the Post-2015 Development period assisted in determining if the world is on course to meet the Sustainable Development Goals, notably goal two, "end hunger, ensure food security and improved nutrition, and promote sustainable agriculture." The interrelation between malnutrition and infections can result in a possibly deadly disease cycle and deterioration of nutritional status. The first 1,000 days of a child's life are critical, and poor nutrition can result in stunted growth, diminished cognitive ability, and poor school and work performance (UNICEF-2020). Undernutrition poses silent crisis in the country. The pervasiveness

6

of underweight children in India is on top globally and is virtually two times of Sub-Saharan Africa. According to the Millennium Development Goal, India is responsible for halving malnourished children's occurrence by 2015.

The consequences of child malnutrition in terms of sickness and death are considerable, and malnutrition has a measurable influence on productivity, therefore failing to invest in tackling malnutrition decreases potential economic growth. The situation is alarming in India with highest prevalence of undernourished children (World Bank, 2015).Protein-energy malnutrition is a state of lack of energy or protein to fulfill the body's metabolic requirements, resulting from either insufficient protein intake and low dietary protein quality, or higher demands due to disease or nutrient depletion. (Mane, V *et al.* 2015).

According to Arunkumar and Hidhathula (2015), undernutrition has a negative impact on cognitive function, motor development, sensory development, and social development. As a result of undernourishment, children would be much less likely positioned to gain from schooling and will earn less as adults.

Bagilkar (2015) described malnutrition as a crucial global health issue because of which millions of children died and are disabled each year. Undernutrition also prevents millions more from reaching their full intellectual and productive potential.

Undernutrition is the main causative factor with a imparing impact on the child's growth, and it also impairs the school recital and efficiency of the child. More than 2 million children died due to malnutrition every year before they reach the age of five. Globally 47.7 per cent of preschoolers are affected with anaemia, and 33.3per cent has vitamin A deficiency (Laillou, A., *et.al*, 2014).

Malnutrition is an important community health marker and fundamental reason for numerous diseases. It is also the foremost factor for the worldwide burden of the disease. It affects one out of three preschool-age children. It has a long-term adverse effect on the physical and cognitive growth of the children. (Dhone *et al.*, 2012).

According to Srivastava *et al.* (2012), undernutrition during preschool age childhood is associated with sluggish cognitive development and severe health impairment later on in life that reduces the superiority of the life of an individual. It is one of the reasons behind the high mortality rates observed in developing countries.

2.2 A Global Scenario of Undernutrition

According to the joint malnutrition statistics, the prevalence of stunting has been dropping since 2000, with more than one in five children stunted under the age of five in 2019, and 47 million suffering from wasting.

According to UNICEF, A very high incidence of stunted population was noticed in three regions in 2019, affecting around one-third of children. On the other hand, three areas showed minimal levels of stunting. However, huge inequalities might exist within locations with lowered down occurrence of stunting. Chronic malnutrition varies greatly between neighbouring nations. About 1 in every 8 people in one state is affected. On the other hand, over one-half of their counterparts in the neighbouring countries, is at a disadvantage because of the irreparable cognitive and physical impairment that can accompany stunted growth.

Stunting affects around 21.3 percent (144 million) of children worldwide, and 6.9 percent (47 million) of children less than five years'. The rate of malnutrition is frightening. Stunting is receding too slowly, whilst wasting continues to have a significant influence on the lives of so many young children. All forms of malnutrition are prevalent in Asia and Africa. Asia and Africa reported that 54% and 40% undernourished children (stunted) <5 years of the age. Asia had 69 percent of the wasted children less than five, and Africa had roughly 27 percent (UNICEF, WHO, World Bank Group Joint malnutrition estimates, 2020 edition).

Around the world, 47 million children under the age of five were found to be malnourished, with 14.3 million of them seriously malnourished. South Asia had more than half of the wasted children and Sub-Saharan Africa had a quarter, with a comparable ratio for seriously wasted children. The 14.8 percent wasting prevalence in South Asia signalled a pressing need for a variety of interventions, including a nutritional programme (UNICEF 2019).

Sultana *et al.* (2019) investigated the prevalence and make out the associated risk aspect of child malnutrition in Bangladesh. 6965 children from 0-59 months of age studied were from 2014 health survey report. The study reported that the incidence of underweight and stunting was 25 percent, and wasting was 11 per cent. The stunting prospect heightened with age and was found the maximum in the children aged 36-37 months. It was extensively higher than children who were less than six months.

8

Berhanu G *et al.* (2018) conducted a community-based comparative cross-sectional study at Albuko district in Ethiopia on preschool children, and the overall results showed that prevalence of stunting children from food-insecure (42.8 per cent) situations outnumber children from food-secure households (35.9 per cent).

Demilew *et al.* (2017) undertook a study on 480 subjects aged 2-3 years' from the slum region of Bahir Dar, Ethiopia. According to the survey, the prevalence of stunting was 42 per cent, underweight was 22.1%, and wasting was 6.4 %. Incidence of severe underweight, wasting, and stunting was respectively 16.3%, 3.8 %, and 1.3%.

Chataut and Khanal (2016) carried out a descriptive study on 402 children less than five years' from rural areas of Kavre, Nepal. Malnourished children made up 7.0 percent of the population, 97 percent were stunted, and 18.9 percent were underweight, according to WHO growth criteria.

Ozor *et al.* (2014) conducted an evocative cross-sectional study on the incidence of undernourishment among children of the age of less than five in Nigeria's Ekpoma community. The research enrolled a number of 402 children. Male children were found to be more prone to be underweight (3.2%) than female children (2.2%). Underweight, stunting, and wasting were found to occur in 2.5, 12.4, and 9.5 percent of the population, respectively.

According to Nisbett et al. (2014), malnutrition have an effect on over 2 billion people worldwide, with roughly 25 percent of all children in low and middle-income nations chronically stunted. The WHO has reported that out of 178 million malnourished children globally, about 20 million are severely malnourished affecting 3.5-5 million death annually among children less than 5years. Furthermore, Asia, particularly south-central Asia, accounts for 70% of the world's wasted (UNICEF-World Bank 2012).

Khambalia *et al.* (2012) analyzed the prevalence and socio-demographic indicators of malnutrition among children in Malaysia. They drew the conclusion that 13.2% of children (0-18 months) were underweight as per Z score. Males were more likely to be underweight than females, and rural children were more affected as compare to urban children.

2.3 A National Scenario of Undernutrition

Singh *et al.* (2019) reviewed a study data of NFHS (2015-16) with seeks to inspect the socioeconomic inequality in malnourished children from 640 districts of India. The study revealed that in India, 38 per cent of children stunted, and 35 percent were underweight. The prevalence of underweight (7 to 67%) and stunting (13 to 65%) children differ significantly across the districts. The districts have a higher contribution of malnourished children to the particular areas of the central-east and West part of the country. The underweight and stunted children were mainly found in the least developed regions of India.

Among the children less than five years, malnutrition status is undoubtedly low compared to global or even South East Asian S.D.G. regions. Further, in some Indian districts, malnutrition is as high as in many other African countries (Chattopadhyay, S .,2019).

Global Hunger (2018) reported that India had been categorized with severe hunger levels in a recent study. Gautam *et al.* (2018) reported the prevalence of stunting of 31.2 per cent and severe stunting of 13.59 per cent among 390 children of Kanpur aged less than five yrs. On the other hand, 14.62 per cent of the children had been found wasted with 6.15 percent cases of severe wasting. The children with mild and moderate malnutrition were 40.51 and 7.95 per cent, respectively, as per the measure of mid-upper arm circumference. A significant correlation between malnutrition and age of the children were also observed.

Vasudevan, & Udayashankar (2019) examined the nutritional level of children of age group less than five years in union territory of Pondicherry and reported that underweight, wasting and stunting in the study area was respectively 18.3 %, 31.6%, and 20.1%. The proportion of moderate and severe underweight and wasting was noticed maximum among 1-2 years age group, whereas, the age group 4-5years had the highest percentage of moderate and severe stunting.

Senthilkumar *et al.* (2018) assessed prevalence of malnutrition and determinants in a group of children less than five years in Coimbatore's tribal area (Tamil Nadu). Overall, 51 per cent of the children were assessed to be undernourished, with 41.3 per cent underweight, of which 11.2 percent were severely malnourished. Nearly 21.8 per cent of children wasted, with 6.8 per cent severely wasted.

Karki *et al.* (2017), performed a study on 390 sample subjects of age 6-59 months to identify the factors and determinants for malnutrition and found that almost half (47.8 percent) of children had a malnourished effect and had no immunization. In contrast, one-fourth (23.26 percent) of the children who were undernourished were vaccinated.

The National Family Health Survey-4 (2015-2016) estimated that in India, every third child under the age of five is underweight, whereas NFHS-3 (2005-2006) estimated that every fifth child found to be underweight.

The records mentioned in ICDS (Integrated Child Development Scheme) centers reported that 27.6 per cent of children of age group 0-6 years that had been enrolled in ICDS centres were found underweight until march 2014 (Demilew, 2017).

The clinical, anthropometric, and biochemical Survey in 2014 (CAB) stated that in Uttar Pradesh the prevalence of stunting among the children was found 62 % that is the highest one. On the other hand the prevalence of underweight and wasting cases was found 45.7 in the district of Jharkhand and 32.4 percent in Chhattisgarh respectively which are the highest percentage of the case. The case of severe stunting is assessed to be elevated in Uttar Pradesh that is 35.6 percent. Whereas, prevalence of severe underweight and severe wasting was found the highest (18.8 % and 11.5%) in Chhattisgarh. Among the district Rai bareli in Uttar Pradesh was found to have the maximum prevalence of the cases of underweight, stunting and wasting that is approximately 77.4 percent. In the state of Uttar Pradesh Hamirpur district and in Bihar, the Aurangabad district was recorded to have the prevalence of 70.2 and 37.2 percent respectively *(*Agarwal.et.al 2018).

2.4 A Regional Scenario of Undernutrition

The prevalence of stunting is not uniformly distributed across the different districts in Haryana. Stunting is comparatively lower in the Mewat district (7%), followed by Karnal and Rewari (17% each), whereas the prevalence of stunting is higher in Kaithal (59 %) and Ambala (48%). Severe stunting is lower in Mewat (3%), followed by Karnal and Panipat (9% each). Overall, 32 percent of the Haryana children belonged to the wasting category, and 19 percent under severe wasting. Variations by districts suggested that wasted children ranged from 19.2 per cent in Mahendargarh to 46 per cent in Karnal. Regions were the ratio of underweight children ranges from 52 per cent in Mewat ("Ministry of Health and Family Welfare DLHS-4).

Jain *et al.* (2018) conducted a study among a sample of 600 children less than five years from a rural region of the Ambala district to assess the nutritional status and the environmental characteristics that affect the children's nutritional status. The study revealed that 30.7 percent of the children were underweight, 7.5 percent wasted and 46.2 percent stunted respectively.

According to a report based on the studies carried out in the districts of Chandigarh, Panchkula, Ambala, Karnal and Yamuna Nagar Children suffer from severe malnutrition. Around 37.4 percent of children in these areas were underweight, while 42.8 percent had stunted growth, and 17.5 per cent were wasting. Nearly all of the children in Karnal, close to 95 per cent, were found to be anaemic. The P.G.I report was published in the daily e-paper D.N.D. (26 March 2014).

NFHS 4 reported that 28.5 percent of children in Haryana were underweight due to chronic and acute malnutrition, followed by 33.4 percent stunted in the urban area and 34.3 per cent in the rural area with 21.3 percent wasted.

According to a report based on a study on the children's nutritional status in Haryana carried out at the district level by Geography and You (2014) for mapping nutritional status, around two-thirds (65.6 percent), were recorded stunted or underweight belonging to 200 odd districts. Estimates further revealed that malnutrition is high (37 per cent) in agriculturally more advanced areas of Karnal, Panipat, Sonipat, Rohtak, and Gurugram.

According to Dr. Rakesh Gupta (2014) of the National Rural Health Mission, children who suffer with acute malnutrition are nine times more likely to die than children being well. Furthermore, malnutrition was responsible for 53 per cent of casualties amongst children less than of five years' in Haryana.

2.5 Undernutrition in preschool children

Osguei (2019) examines the association between demographic status, socio-economic status and nutritional level of Nepalese children < five yrs. A study of 3630 children found that 46.3 percent were stunted, 38.1 percent were underweight, 14.1 percent were wasted, and 44.9 percent were anaemic.

In a cross-sectional study on 600 children in district Rohtak's rural areas among children of 1-5 years of age, nearly 41.3 per cent of subjects were found stunted and

12

54.4 per cent were malnourished. The prevalence of underweight and stunting was more among girls (Gupta *et al.* 2019).

Nayak *et al.* (2018) conducted a community-based case study among preschool children of 3-6 years attending Anganwadi centers of Udupi, district of Karnataka, India. The majority (45.8%) of the children belonged to the 3-4 yrs of age group. The maximum (84.4%) of the children were in low socioeconomic status and were underweight. Undernutrition and the socioeconomic status of the parents was observed significantly associated.

Bharati, (2018) studied the growth and the impact of socioeconomic variables on preschool children nutritional status. 205935 children aged 0-59 months, showed a progressive development in all the age groups. The proportion of underweight boys was highest for the 9 and 23 months as compared to 12-35 months old girls. The large ratio of underweight or stunted children progressed from 6 months to the next second year of life.

A study of 400 preschool children of rural areas of Chhattisgarh state reported prevalence of 36% of underweight, 35.5 % stunted, and rest 28.5 % were under the category of wasting. Nearly half of the girl children were found to be malnourished and stunted. The proportion of female children was more nutritionally destitute than males (Sukla and Borkar, 2018). A study was carried out with the thirty slums of Kanpur cluster sampling each cluster having 390 children aged 0-60 months, and the result based on WHO classification indicated the prevalence of stunting (31.28%) and severe Stunting (13.59%). The wasting subjects were categorized in two, i.e., wasting (14.62 %) and severe wasting (6.15%). As per the mid-upper arm circumference criteria, moderate malnutrition was 40.59 percent and 7.97 per cent were severely malnourished. The finding further concluded that malnutrition's prevalence decreased significantly with better maternal education (Gautam. 2018).

Karki *et al.* (2017) examined a study with underweight children under the age of five in Nepal and concluded that one-quarter (26.16 percent) of the children were mildly malnourished based on MUAC (mid-upper arm circumference).

A study on children aged 1-7 yrs aged children, conducted in governmental and non-governmental kindergartens in Kosovo, revealed that the average for WAZ, HAZ and

WHZ were all within 0.0 and 0.1. A proportion of stunted children was 1.3per cent, while the proportion of wasting children was 1.9 per cent (Rysha,*et.al.* 2017).

A study on 456 preschool children of 3-6 years participated in Anganwadi centers in Kannur district, Kerala, explained 17.3 percent underweight prevalence and a significant association between the nutritional status It was also determined that mother's level of education is important in preventing underweight in preschool children S.S,Anitha *et al.* (2017).

Pasha Mushtaq *et al.* (2017), performed a pilot cross-sectional research in Nandayal, Andhra Pradesh, to evaluate the nutritional status and stratify the effects involved with preschool children's nutritional status. There were a total of 161 children aged 3-6 years, with 42.2% and 57.8 % respectively males and females. Malnourished children in the second degree (according to the Gomez classification) accounted for 47.8 percent of the total, with the first degree accounting for 39.1 percent. The study also discovered that the mother's education and socioeconomic status had an additional impact on the second and first degrees of undernutrition.

Saaka and Zackaria (2016) assessed the relationship between wasting and stunting on 2,720 preschool children of Ghanania. The incidence of simultaneous wasting and stunting within and between children aged less than 5 yrs was lesser i.e. at 1.4 percent. Children with low weight-for-height scores had a higher risk of linear stunted growth (stunting), particularly those under the age of three.

Islam *et.al.* (2014) carried out a descriptive study with 144 under-five children from Tangail's rural and urban areas (72 children each). Weight-for-height study reflected that children found to be severely wasted were 1.39 percent, moderately wasted (1.39 percent), and mildly wasted (22.23 percent) in the rural area. Weight-for-age results showed that children were relatively underweight (38.8 percent mild and 25 percent moderately malnourished), and the preponderance of height-for-age among rural children was 44.45 percent higher than among urban children (2.7 per cent). The study further concluded that nutritional knowledge, personal hygiene practices, breastfeeding, adding nutritious value-added food, community education, and dietary patterns would significantly improve the children's nutritional status.

2.6 The role of probiotic in enhancing the nutritional status of undernourished children

A research was conducted on the iron deficient children with interventiom of probiotics before and after test. One group of children was supplemented with iron syrup and other group was intervened with iron syurp with fermented milk containing fructo-oligosaccharides and lactobacillusplantarum for 90 days. The result revealed that serum ferritin, haemoglobin level and body weight, height of the children increased significantly ($p \leq 0.05$) who were intervened with fermented milk and iron syrup (Helmyati et.al.2020).

Synbiotic (probiotic and prebiotic bacteria) supplementation effects on the growth of children between the age of 2-5 years, selected from the Khatamolanbia Clinic, Shahid Sadoughi University of Medical Sciences, Yazad, Iran were investigated sixty-nine FTT (Failure to thrive) patients were involved and the study showed that out of 69 patients, 81 per cent were mild underweight, and the remaining 19 per cent were of moderate underweight. The patients were introduced with probiotic and prebiotic bacteria for a month. The mean weight of the children in the symbiotic group increased significantly. The study also suggested that symbiotic can be effective in weight and BMI gain, especially in undernourished children (Aflatoonia et al., 2020).

Onubi et al. (2015) discussed the advantages of consuming prebiotics (produced by probiotics) in terms of weight and height gain, particularly in malnourished children in developing countries. Furthermore, the children's growth curves in the probiotic groups were considerably higher than others in the comparison group, implying that probiotics aid in the compensatory growth of children with stunting.

Famouri et al. (2014) undertook a triple-blinded research in Shahrekord, Iran to study the effects of synbiotic on children's growth. A total of 84 underweight children aged 12 to 54 months, 42 each in both the groups (control and supplemented), and the children who were selected for study were assigned as interventional and control groups. The interventional group was intervened with synbiotic and starch powder in a sachet, containing 150 million spore bacillus coagulants and 100 mg fructo-oligosaccharides for six months. Results showed significant increasing effect on the weight of interventional group.

Surono et.al. (2014) conducted a ninety-day randomised, double-blind study on

15

Indonesian children aged 12-24 months. There were four categories (Placebo, probiotic, zinc supplementation, and a combination of probiotics and zinc). The results showed a good prospective to improve children's zinc levels after taking a combination of probiotic L. and plantarum IS-1056 and zinc supplementation in the experiment, as well as a significantly improved humoral immune response.

Protective effects of probiotics and their impact on preschool children aged 2-5 years living in urban slums with a sample of 379 preschool children were assessed by Hemalatha *et.al* (2014). The Children were intervened in three randomly allocated groups with probiotics for nine months to estimate weight gain and their effect on linear growth, diarrhoea and fever and it was found that it helped to make a healthy gut.

A double-blind, randomized pre-post trial study was carried out for 90 days on the preschool children of Indonesia to measure the effects of the probiotic, on the body weight, or the humoral immune response, with two groups (placebo and probiotic). Total serum & salivary levels were analyzed along with the children's body weight measurement. The total serum did not extensively increase in the probiotic group than the placebo group. In contrast, the whole salivary level and the children's body weight increased significantly ($p \leq 0.05$) in the probiotic group compared to the placebo group. The salivary level was substantially more in underweight children who intervened with probiotics. The study additionally found that probiotics had positive effects on weight gain, total salivary level, and humoral immune response in underweight children (Surono *et al*. 2011).

Sazawal (2010) also assessed the consumption of probiotics and prebiotic milk for one year resulted in an increase in weight gain and iron content in the body of experimental children from Sangam Vihar, New Delhi.

2.7 Development and sensory evaluation of Value-added food preparations

Zegeye *et al*. (2019) formulated cookies from the blended flour of sorghum and wheat added with soybean flour, and the preparations indicated a significant increase in ash and fat. Organoleptic acceptability was based on color, taste, flavor, texture, appearance, and crunchiness. It was illustrated that soybean and sorghum could be effectively supplemented with wheat at 5 per cent sorghum and 10 per cent soybean to provide overall acceptability. The incorporation of wheat and sorghum blend in the flour up to 20 per cent provided cookies satisfactory acceptable organoleptic superiority.

Srivastava, (2017) planned a study to develop fortified food products by adding spirulina in noodles, cookies, and pasta to improve nutrient contents (protein, calcium, iron, copper, phosphorous, and vitamin B12) in the food products. Adding spirulina in pasta and noodles at 5 and at 10 percent in biscuits was most acceptable on sensory evaluation indicators. The study's outcome revealed that the developed food preparations were quite nutritious. The nutritional value was comparatively higher than the control group, and fortified food products using spirulina help combat malnutrition.

Adegoke *et al.* (2017) evaluated the acceptability of various food preparations that formulate turmeric powder, soybean flour, and wheat flour. The optimal flour blend used to develop the biscuit consisted of turmeric powder, of ratio 0.5 percent, and soybean flour, 26.63 per cent, with wheat flour 72.88 per cent, respectively. The sensory evaluation compared with control (100 % refined wheat four) revealed a significant effect at the level of 5 per cent.

Pasupuleti *et al.* (2017) conducted a study to assess krishna poshak mix *laddus'* given efficacy on the nutritional status of 100 preschool children (50 experimental & 50 control) in rural areas of Guntur District of Andhra Pradesh. The results indicated that supplemented *Krishna Poshak* mix *laddus* to the children is an efficient supplement to improve the children's anthropometric measurement. The primary analysis suggested mean weight gain as 12.7±1.07, and UMAC was13.16±1.09. After six weeks of the intervention, the calculated mean weight was 13.31±1.10, and UMAC was 13.6±0.7.

Ingle and Nawkar (2016) discovered that supplementing soy flour in wheat flour at four levels, i.e., 10, 15, 20, and 25 % for value-added food preparation, resulted in sensory attributes ranging from 6.9 to 8.1. The lower sensory score of 25 per cent was observed, claiming that a higher amount of soy flour reduces the sensory parameters. The most acceptable level was at 20 percent. The proximate composition of food preparations fortified with 10 percent skimmed milk powder contained a better percentage of protein, i.e.16.2– 21.1 per cent, carbohydrates (67.66-77.2 per cent), fat (1.9-4.5 per cent), fiber (1.22-1.73 per cent) and ash (0.7-1.42 per cent). The study concluded that soy flour fortification might be considered excellent in protein with a good scope of acceptability.

Baniwal and Grewal (2015), in order to formulate a cereal-pulse mixture as a ready-to-eat snack, with proximate composition (total dietary fiber and minerals), conducted a trial and assessed for different cereal flours (maize & wheat) and the pulse flour (soybean and green gram) and a controlled snack from the wheat flour and maize grits mixture was used. The snack blend formulated from the alternate wheat–maize mixture with 15 per cent pulse flour scored maximum nutritional quality & overall acceptability. The trial suggested that the pulse (soybean and green gram) could be gainfully utilized to make value-added snacks.

Nkesiga and Gabriel. (2015) planned a trial to evaluate the effects of amaranth leaf flour on the proficient, chemical and sensory attributes of extrudates from flour blends of soybean and yellow maize. Amarnath leaf flour was added into yellow maize and soybean (70:30) combined with flour at five different levels, i.e., 0, 5, 10, 15, and 20 per cent to develop snacks and control groups 100 per cent wheat flour. Addition of soyabean flour & amaranth leaf significantly (p<0.05) increased the energy level (349.72 to 360.07), protein (17.88 to 21.67), minerals, and vitamin content as compared to control. The most acceptable was assessed as the control (wheat flour). On the other hand, snacks' acceptability reduced with increasing extra amaranth leaf flour. Incorporation of amaranth leaf at 10 per cent was comparatively better acceptable.

Farzana and Mohajan (2015) intended to assess the quality attributes of formulating soy-mushroom supplemented baked goods with wheat flour replaced by enriched flour at three levels, like 10, 15, and 20 per cent. The control biscuits were made without soy flour, but mushroom powder was added to both preparations. An organoleptic evaluation and chemical estimation addition of 15 per cent soy flour resulted in favourable scores. When compared to the control, the energy content of soy flour supplemented baked goods enhanced to 463-485 Kcal/g, with a significant increase in protein (11.07 to 17.86%), fat (17.36 to 20.89%), iron (1.56 to 1.99 mg/g), and fibre (0.45 to 0.92 per cent).

De Marco et al. (2014), a trial was carried out a trial to estimate the effects of adding spirulina on dried pasta's technological and nutritional quality attributes. Wheat flour was substituted by spirulina at three different levels, i.e., 5g, 10g, and 20g. In contrast, the control (without spirulina) sample was compared and analyzed for its technical and nutritional quality characteristics and the technical quality was analyzed in terms of cooking behavior and texture profile. Besides, it has also been subjected to its measurement of protein content, *in Vitro* phenolic compound, antioxidant activity, and protein digestibility. It was pointed out that the addition of spirulina in pasta has shown an increase in antioxidant properties and a good amount of protein content as compared to control. The pasta with 20gram of spirulina considerably altered technological quality characteristics.

Ndif. *et al.* (2014) developed biscuits by introducing full-fat soy flour at different levels with wheat flour and inferred that the cookies were well acceptable at 30 and 50 percent of the addition of soy flour with wheat flour.

Bansal and Kochhar (2013) incorporated peanut flour in traditional recipes at a level of 5-50 per cent. They found it to be highly acceptable and recommended to improve the nutritional status of the diets.

Vijayarani *et al.* (2012) analyzed the sensory evaluation of the developed value-added product (pasta) incorporating spirulina, prepared at four different levels where one was considered as control. The spirulina level was 5, 10, and 15 per cent, respectively. It was inferred that 5 per cent spirulina incorporated pasta had a maximum mean score.

2.8 Role of feeding interventions in improving nutritional status of children

Castro *et al.* (2017, conducted trials on 110 preschool children aged 2-5 years in Brazil to measure the effects of vitamin and mineral product supplemented inulin (a prebiotic fiber) on vitamin A and iron status of children. 30 g of inulin diluted in 100ml of water, supplemented five times a week, given daily for 45 days. It was inferred that values of Z scores and all parameters were significantly higher after the intervention. The supplementation significantly improved the intake level of energy, micro, and macro-nutrients and improved the iron and anthropometric status of the product developed.

Matondo *et al.* (2016) conducted trial to evaluate the nutritional status of 50 malnourished children aged 6 to 60 from the center de "Nutrition Therapeutique of Kisantu" Congo. All the children were found to be anaemic (20 per cent of children were severely anaemic and 80 per cent were moderate anaemic), WAZ.and HAZ. Scores revealed that 78 per cent and 84 per cent of the study population were affected by acute malnutrition in the study area. In contrast, edema was found in 64 per cent of the sample subjects. The two groups were formed with one as control and another as an intervention group. The intervention group children received 10 grams of spirulina powder per day (5g in the morning and 5g in the evening) with their daily local diet. The height, weight, hemoglobin, albumin, red blood cell count, and hematocrit were measured before and after completing the experiment. The results showed a significant increase in hemoglobin level and hematocrit levels of the children in the treatment group in comparison to the control group, the anaemia level decreased from 20 per cent to 6 per cent, and edema cut down from 64 per cent to 4 percent at the end of the study.

The impact of developed spirulina fortified biscuits on two anaemic groups (experimental and control group) was assessed at Allahabad's. The analysis result shows that the biscuits contained 2.55 per cent moisture, 6.25 per cent protein, 20.43 per cent fat, 1.18 per cent crude fiber, 4.07 per cent ash, 2.88.98 per cent calcium, 115.92 per cent phosphorus, and 3.94 per cent iron. Developed fortified biscuits intervened to the subjects for 45 days resulted into a significant increase in hemoglobin level (1.66g/dl) than the control group (Fatima and Srivastava,2016).

Prasad *et al.* (2016) conducted a trial to develop nutrient-specific, digestible, and economically ready-to-eat supplementary food, i.e., *seviyan, pinni, panjiri, mathi*, and biscuits, were prepared from sprouted cereal & pulse along with standardized spinach leaves or potato flour. Tukey's test was used to estimate different sensory evaluation scores within varying levels of treatments. All the developed supplementary food was acceptable at 30 percent with potato flour and 2.5 per cent of spinach powder. The mean scores of ready-to-eat complementary foods differed significantly (p<0.05).The addition of a variety of supplemental food helps to enhance malnourished children's nutritional status.

Steenkamp. *et al.*(2015) planned a study on children with moderate acute malnutrition (12-60 months). The research study was made to determine the anthropometric alteration in those who were intervened with ready to use supplementary food for six weeks, followed up until 12 weeks. The Z-scores for weight-for-age, height-for-age, weight-for-height, and mid-upper arm circumference, all improved significantly.

Maximum (70.5%) of the subjects stood in a similar malnutrition classification, and only 26 per cent recovered. The children's growth rate with a low initial weight-for-height was found significantly higher, i.e., r = -0.15, p<0.05, followed by those with less wasting.

An experiment was carried out on 54 children from Anganwadi of the Malakpur district of Satara Maharashtra aged 3-5 years to assess the effectiveness of the supplemented *Krishna Poshak* mix on the children's nutritional status. The experimental group was intervened with KPS mix *laddus,* whereas the control group allowed ICDS supplementary diet. The mean value of pre and post-weight (13.61 and 14.08) of and mid-arm circumference (14.90 and 15.14), the children in the experimental group were comparatively higher than that control. The significant gain of weight and mid-arm circumference. It was concluded that *laddus* played a vital role in improving children's nutritional status (Mulik and Salunkhe 2014).

Amegovu *et al.* (2014) planned a single-blind randomized study trial with 392 children of 6-59 months of age from Karamoja, Uganda, on the efficacy of sorghum peanut blend and corn-soy blend on moderate acute malnutrition treatment. The sorghum peanut blend mixed with honey and ghee was in contrast to the corn-soy mixture with added sugar and vegetable oil, the combination (CSB+ or S.P.B.) given to every subject for a pair of three months. The improvement velocity was not significantly distinct for the CSB+ group (82.3%) or the S.P.B. group (76.8%), chi-square test P= 0.093.

Douamba *et al.* (2012), undertook a study on 304 malnourished children aged (6-48) months in order to estimate the impacts of a cereal and soy dietary preparation on the health parameters of undernourished children in Ouagadougou, Burkina Faso. Children (172 female and 132 male) were intervened with developed value-added food (composed of 60 per cent of small millet, 20 per cent of soybean, and 10 per cent of groundnuts). It was inferred that after of the intervention 63.81 per cent of children improved with the normal W.H.Z.> −2. Result showed that, there were only 6.58 per cent children with W.H.Z. <−3.

2.9 Impact of nutrition education and counselling

Fadare *et al.* (2019), in their investigation, reported that mother's knowledge had positive & optimistic link with weight-for-height and height-for-age Z scores in the children. A mother with a higher level of education possesses a momentous positive involvement with the child's height-for-age and weight-for-height Z scores. Hence, imparting nutrition education and knowledge to mothers is a vital footer to bring into better nutrition status.

Oly-Alawuba et al. (2017) also revealed in their study a significant ($p \leq 0.05$) change on correlation between the mother's nutrition knowledge and anthropometric parameters among 400 children aged 2-5 years.

Sharma and Lakhawat (2017) conducted the pre and post-test before and after imparting education to mothers. The baseline (pre-test) scores of all the mothers expressed a low level of nutrition knowledge. After imparting nutrition education, a maximum (82%) of mothers gained a high level of nutrition awareness. The study also found that 39.8 percent of the subjects were familiar with food, but this increased to 75 percent after imparting nutrition education. The knowledge regarding the food groups illustrated at the primary level was only 7.5 per cent, which improved to 77.5 percent afterwards. Mothers had poor knowledge (4.7%) about nutrition deficiency diseases; however, it increased (82.1%) after gaining nutrition education.

 A short-term training program was conducted to evaluate the knowledge of forty-five mothers of under-five children and to measure the effect of pre-arranged training instructions in a backward region of New Delhi. The pre-test proportion of 40 per cent of mothers had poor knowledge, 33.3 per cent had average knowledge, and only 26.7 per cent possessed better knowledge. On the other hand, post-test scores suggested that only 26.7 percent had poor knowledge, 46.7 percent acquired average knowledge, and the rest- 26.7 percent gained adequate knowledge (Mishra. et al. 2017).

Sahana and Chandrasekhar (2016), conducted a study on the mothers of children under five groups from Shimoga, Karnataka, and concluded that more than half (55.2% and 55.8%) of the children were underweight and stunted whose mothers were illiterate as compared to the children of mothers who possessed primary education (41.0% and 42.9%). The children of the mothers who were employed were weak with stunting and underweight (77.4% and 80.6%) compared to home wives, i.e., 46.8 percent and 48.0 percent, respectively.

Priyanka and Veenu (2015) also assessed impact of nutrition education on mothers' nutritional knowledge. The pre-scores exemplify a lack of nutrition knowledge in mothers in the study area. The post-scores had a significant (p<0.01) gain in knowledge after imparting nutrition education.

Aparna (2015) evaluates the consistency and efficiency of designed nutrition education programs to spread awareness concerning PEM (protein-energy malnutrition) amongst the mothers of children aged less than five. Results have shown a significant (p≤0.05) growth in mothers' knowledge compared to pre-test scores.

Sengupta and S Benjamin (2014) conducted a community-based intercession study on a sample of 101 children of 2-5 years from an urban slum area of Ludhiana on the impact of mother education and motivation. The nutritional and health education was provided to increase their knowledge and educate them to prepare various types of low-cost healthy supplemented food for their children.

Singh and Babu (2013) conducted a trial on 412 primary school children in Hyderabad. The study concluded underweight children were 28.9 per cent and 21.8 per cent were found stunted, and a higher percentage was observed in children of illiterate parents.

Shettigar et al. (2013) conducted a cross-sectional descriptive research on 50 mothers with children under the age of five in rural Kotekar (Mangalore) to assess their knowledge of nutritional problems. Nearly half of the mothers (54%) had poor knowledge, around 38 per cent average, and only 8 per cent had good knowledge.

John (2011) conducted a study on 500 preschool children aged 3-6 years of the tsunami-affected region of district Nagapattinam. It was noticed that maximum children were undernourished, and a significant difference was observed between mean nutrient intake and RDA. The difference between the pre-test and the post-test mean value was significant (p≤0.01).

According to Ramrao (2013), the most of the adolescent girls evaluated either have low or fair awareness and knowledge about women's healthcare and dietary habits. After two months of training in reproductive health care and nutritional awareness, their awareness and behaviours improved significantly, and their percentage scores increased significantly. Nutrition education had shown a good sign in increasing the level of nutrition knowledge and nutrient intake before and after imparting nutrition education. However Kaur, 2007 observed significant increase in energy, protein, carbohydrates, and all the vitamins except vitamin B_{12} and minerals increased (P $\leq$0.01) significantly.

Yusoff Hofzan *et al.* (2012) discovered that nutrition education could effectively increase knowledge, behaviours, and haemoglobin levels among Malaysian secondary school adolescents. When nutrition education is appropriately focused on behaviour, it is most effective.

CHAPTER - 3

MATERIALS AND METHODS

In this chapter, the necessary outlines of the planning of the experiment will be discussed in a very systematic order. On the other hand, the research investigation's execution part is thoroughly discussed in Chapter 4.

Statement of the problem:

Enriched food and education to combat Child Malnutrition

3.1 Phase I: Pre-intervention

3.1.1 Site of the study

3.1.2 Domain of the study

3.1.3 Selecting of samples

3.1.4 Designing and pretesting of questionnaire-cum-interview schedule

3.1.5 Collection of data

3.1.6 Assessment of nutritional status

    3.1.6.1 Anthropometric measurement

    3.1.6.2 Clinical assessment

    3.1.6.3 Biochemical assessment

    3.1.6.4 Dietary assessment

3.1.7 Preparation of education material and evaluation of nutritional knowledge level

3.1.8 Developed enriched food preparations for interventions.

3.2 Phase II: Intervention Phase

3.3 Phase III: Post-Intervention Phase

3.4 Statistical Analysis

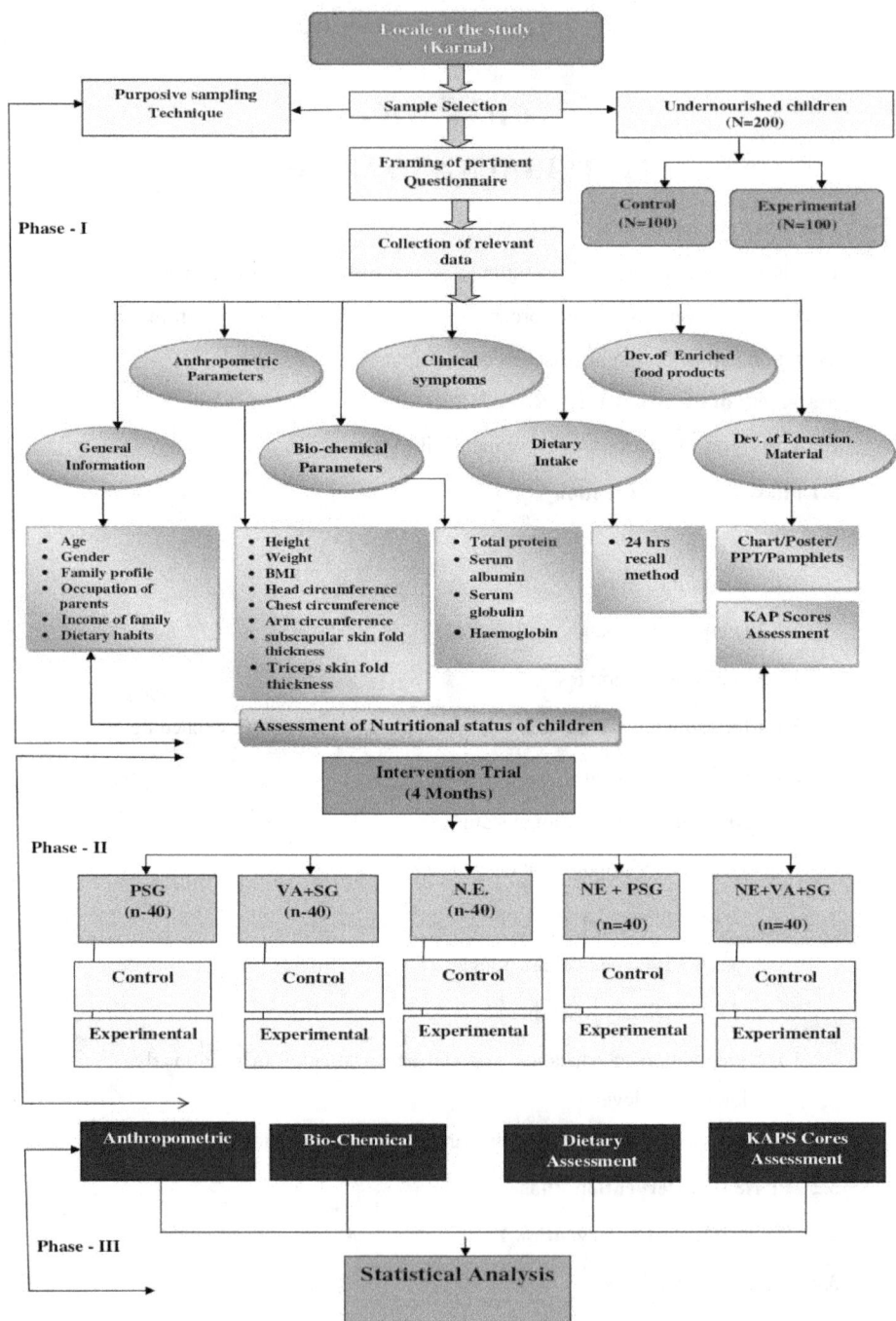

Fig.3.1 Plan of Study

3.1 Phase I: Pre-intervention

3.1.1 Site of the study:

Karnal district was purposively selected for the study.

3.1.2 Domain of the study:

Ghadaria Mohalla, Sadar, Ghasaria Mohalla, Valmiki Colony, Bakara Mohalla, Drabi line, Bheem Nagar, and jhugis near sector 12

3.1.3 Selecting of samples:

A group of 200 undernourished children between the ages of 3 and 6 years' randomly selected from the area the domain as prescribed above constituted the basis of the study. Purposively selected of 200, under-nourished children were further stratified according to the experiment plan and grouped into five groups. It is also specified that each of the five groups were further sub-grouped into experimental and controlled groups as per the research requirement and is presented in the following paragraph.

3.1.4 Designing and pretesting of questionnaire-cum-interview schedule:

A self-constructed and pretested interview schedule was prepared to be introduced to parents to obtain the basic information on the family concerning age, gender, initial weight and height, education status of the parents and also the parent's occupation status, family type, house type, annual income, eating and dietary habits of the children. All the questions and content was standardized in consultation with the supervisor, senior faculty of sister department and some experts in the field of specialization.

3.1.5 Collection of data:

Personal visits were made to interview the parents to collect relevant information with the help of the interview schedule as finalized above. The data so collected on age, gender, initial weight & height, education status of the parents, parents' occupation status, family type, house type, annual income, eating, and dietary habits of the children were subjected to further tabulation and analysis leading to logical and scientific inferences.

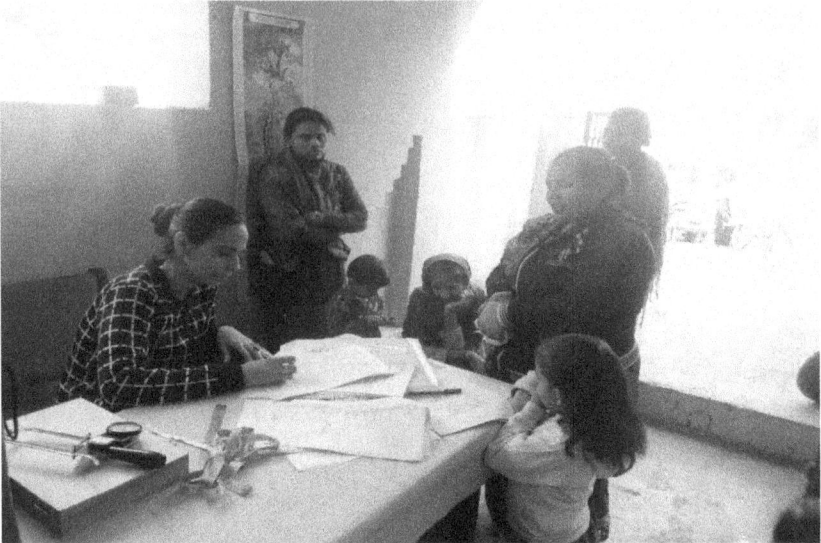

COLLECTING INFORMATION

3.1.6 Assessment of Nutritional Status:

Nutritional status refers to a person's state of health and it was propelled through intake and consumption of the nutrients. Methods that pertained to measuring the nutritional status of the subjects were as follows:

3.1.6.1 Anthropometric measurement:

An anthropometric measure generally refers to the measurements of body size. It's a quantitative method that would be intensely susceptible to nutritional status amongst children. It is widely recognized as one of the valuable techniques to detect undernutrition (NIN, 2010). The following parameters were measured:

i. **Measurement of Height:** The height of the children was measured using the technique of "Jelliffe (1966)". The vertical height was measured by rod hooked up to the platform employed. The children were positioned barefoot, head one straight, comfortably erect with straight back and shoulders relaxed against the vertical measuring rod, and then measurements were recorded at the nearest 0.1cm (WHO 2006).

28

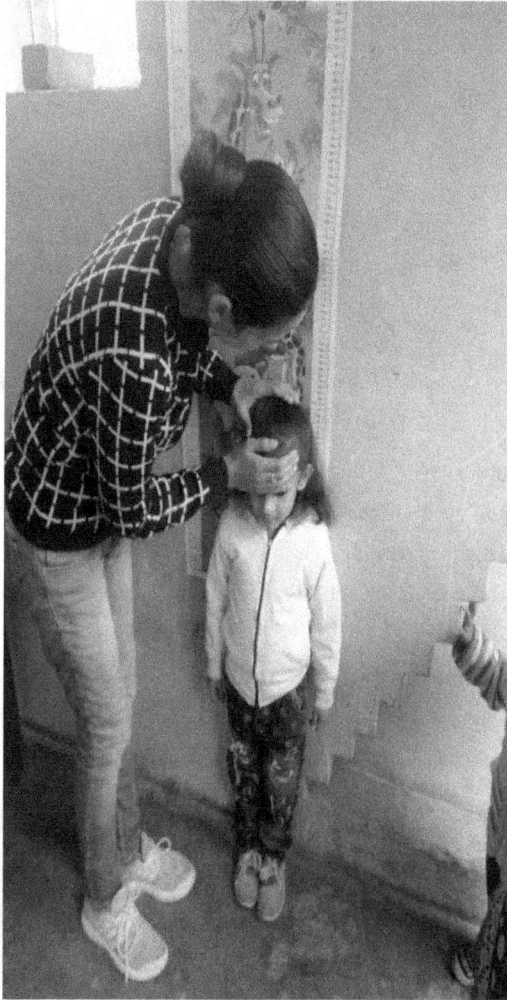

HEIGHT MEASUREMENT

ii.   **Measurement of weight:** Weight (kg) was measured with a spring hanging scale (Salter) with a precision of 0.1kg (100g). The Salter hung to the roof and the child was placed in the weighing pants, and then hooked the pants to the scale. When the Salter stabled, then the weight was recorded to the nearest 100g. The child hangs freely without holding onto anything.

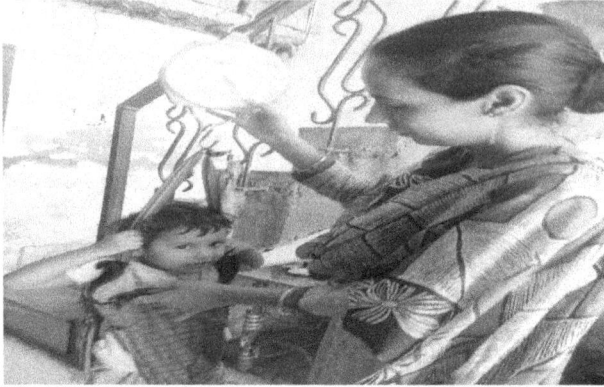

WEIGHT MEASUREMENT

iii.   **Head circumference:** A flexible, non-stretchable narrow tape (less than 1 cm wide) was employed to measure the head circumference. The measurement has been recorded at the nearest 0.1cm.

iv.   **Chest circumference:** The chest circumference was measured at the nipple line level in mid-inspiration with a flexible, non-stretchable tape made of fiber glass.

v.   **Mid upper arm circumference (MUAC):** A narrow, flexible, and non-stretchable shakir tape had been used and MUAC was measured, placing the tape around the middle part of the child's left upper arm.

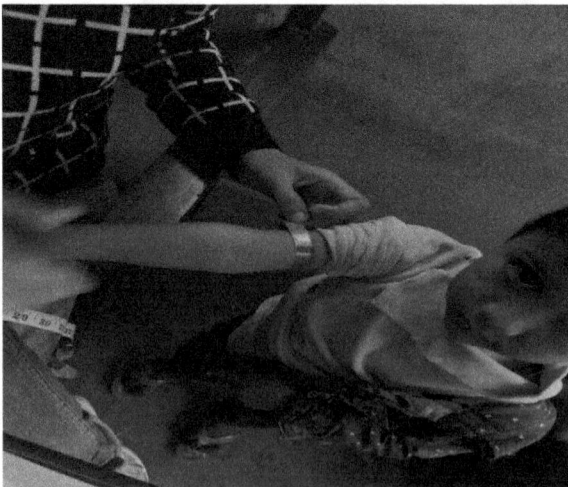

MUAC MEASUREMENT

vi. **Skin fold measurement:** Harpenden Skin fold caliper had been employed to measure skin fold thickness (over the triceps and subscapular region).

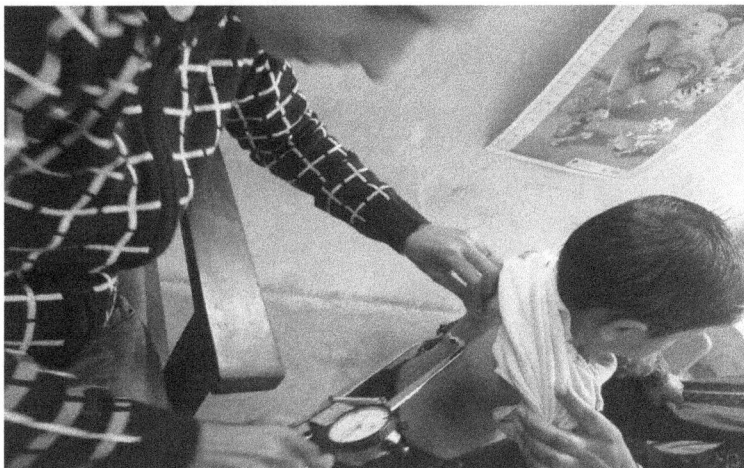

SUBSCAPULAR SKINFOLD THICKNESS MEASUREMENT

vii. **Z-score classification:** The nutritional status of the children was evaluated, categorizing weight and height according to z-scores. The z-scores for different indicators like "weight-for-age, height-for-age, and BMI-for-age" (weight-for height) were calculated using "WHO anthroplus software" (Zuguo and Laurence 2007). The prevalence of malnutrition was estimated based on the z-score cut-off level of WHO (2006) given below:

Table 3.1 Prevalence of malnutrition using standard z-score classification (WHO, 2006)

z-score cut-off level	Grade of malnutrition
> +2.0 SD	Overweight
-2.0 SD to +2SD	Normal
<-2.0 SD	Moderately malnourished
<-3.0SD	Severely malnourished

3.1.6.2 Clinical assessment: Observation about the general appearance of a child's hair, eye, lips, tongue, teeth, gums, nails, skin, and appearance has been taken under the guidance and supervision of medical staff.

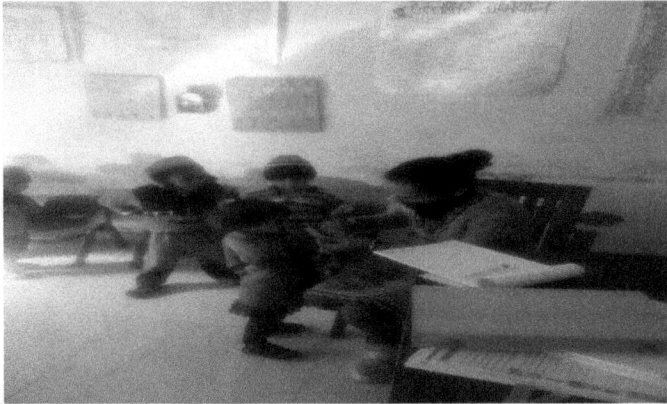

CLINICAL ASSESSMENT

3.1.6.3 Biochemical assessment: Biochemical assessment was done at pre, during, and post-intervention stages. For analysis, 2ml of the blood sample was acquired from each subject by a well-trained and experienced lab technician using a 5 ml disposable syringe (Dispovan). Blood samples were examined in Shri Guru Singh Sabha Charitable lab Karnal to analyze hemoglobin, total protein, serum albumin, and serum globulin.

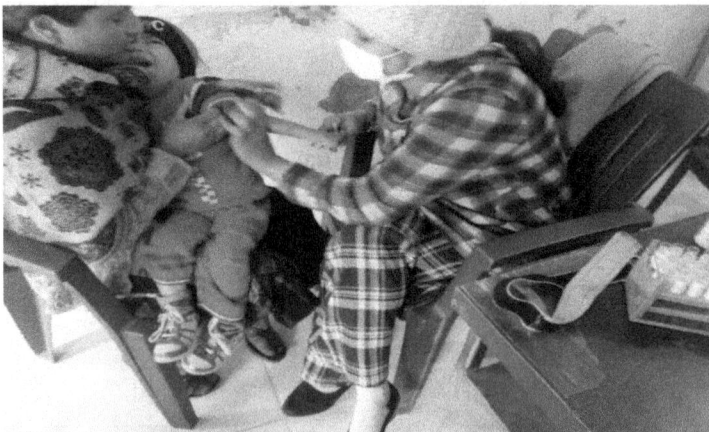

BLOOD SAMPLE COLLECTION

a) Hemoglobin determination: "The Sysemex XE-2100 hematology automated analyzer was used to get a rapid complete full blood count. The Sysemex XE-2100 employs three detector blocks and two kinds of reagents for blood analysis. The WBC count was measured by the WBC detector block using the D.C. detection method, and the R.B.C. count was measured by the R.B.C. detector block using the D.C. detection method. The H.G.B. detector block measured the hemoglobin concentration using the non-cyanide hemoglobin method."

Principle: "3.0 µL of blood sample diluted first, dilute the sample to the ratio 1:33 using cell pack with 0.99970 ml .dispensed beforehand in containers, and then moves through a thin tube so that cell pass by one at a time, cells were measured using fluorescence flow cytometry. It can run on its own. 0.5 ml of 'Sulfolyser added into the R.B.C. and hemoglobin converted into S.L.S. hemoglobin (to formulate 1.500 diluted samples). As the tubes go through the machine, two are picked up and inverted five times to mix. The first on sampled they put down again, the rack moves along one space, and two more are picked up and mixed five times; this assures that each tube is inverted ten times before being sampled."

"The caps are left on the tubes as they go through the machine. A piercer takes a sample through the rubber center while the tube is upside down. EDTA (lavender) tube is by and large used, although citrate (blue top) tubes will also work (although the result must correct because of dilution). The wavelength of 555nm surpassed throughout the lens to the sample in the haemoglobin cells."

Reagents:

i.   Stromatolyser Solution

ii.   Diluent Solution

Table 3.2*Classification of anaemia

The severity of anemia based on hemoglobin	Hemoglobin level (g/dl)
Non- anaemic	>11.5
Anemic	11.5
Mild	10-11.5
Moderate	7-10
Severe	<7

*Source Nation Institute of Nutrition (NIN 1986)

b) Total Protein Estimation: Total protein level in blood may increase mainly due to dehydration or decrease due to various deficiencies, including malnutrition. "The total protein of the subjects was calculated by the Biuret method."

Principle: "Protein and peptides, similarly to biuret, react with cupric ions (Cu^{2+}) in alkaline solutions to form a violet complex suitable for photometric determination."

Procedure: "Mix well and incubate at 37°C for 10 min or at R.T. for 30min. Measure the standard (Abs.S) absorbance and Test sample (Abs.T) against the blank 60min."

Addition Sequence	Blank (ml)	Standard (ml)	Test (ml)
Biuret reagent (L1)	1.0	1.0	1.0
Distilled water	0.02	-	-
Protein standard (S)	-	0.02	-
Sample	-	-	0.02

Calculation: Total Protein Concentration (g/dl) = Abs.T × 8

Abs.S

Measure the absorbance of the sample and the standard at 550 nm against the blank.

Table 3.3 Reference values for Total Protein Level among children

Total Protein	Total protein level (g/dl)
Normal	6.0-8.3
Moderate	5.9-3.9
Low	>3.9

C) Serum Albumin Estimation: Serum albumin level is an index to assess protein nutritional status in children. Serum albumin was calculated by in vitro diagnostic kit used for quantitative determination.

Principle: "Albumin in buffered solution reacts with the anionic bromocresol green (B.C.G.) with a dye-binding reaction to give a proportionate green color, which should measure at 628nm (600-650nm). The final color is stable for 10 minutes."

Reagent 1(Bromocresol Green):

Succinic Acid 94mmol/L

Sodium Hydroxide 10.2mmol/L

BCG 0.149mmol/L

Standard (albumin 5g/L):

B.S.A. 50g/L

Procedure: The samples and the reagent were brought to room temperature before use.

	Blank	Standard	Test
Reagent 1	1ml	1ml	1ml
Standard	-	10μL	-
Sample	-	-	10μL

Incubate for 1 minute at room temperature. Mix and read.

Calculation: "Sample Concentration (g/dl) = Abs.of Sample –Abs. of Blank × 5

Abs. of standard- Abs. of Blank"

Table 3.4 Reference values of Serum Albumin Levels among children

Serum Albumin Status	Serum albumin level (g/dl)
Acceptable (Low risk)	>3.5
Low (moderate risk)	2.8- 3.4
Deficient (high risk)	<2.8

d) Serum Globulin Estimation: Serum globulin level drops due to decreased synthesis, inherited immune deficiency, and malnutrition. The method used to determine serum globulin:

Calculation: Globulin = Total protein – albumin

Table 3.5 Reference values of Serum Globulin Levels among children

Serum Globulin Status	Serum globulin level (g/dl)
Acceptable (Low risk)	<2.6
Low (moderate risk)	1.8-2.5
Deficient (high risk)	>1.8

3.1.6.4 Dietary assessment:

a) **Dietary habits and dietary intake:** The dietary evaluation was done for three consecutive days using the "24-hour recall method". Information regarding dietary habits, likes and dislikes of food, meal intake, preference for various food, and dietary intake was fetched. Food groups included were roots and tubers, green leafy vegetables, other vegetables, cereals, pulses, fruit, sugar and jaggery, milk and milk products and fat and oils.

b) **Food Intake:** The food intake was recorded using standardized utensils, shown to the children's mother to let them know the amount of food consumed by children. The information collected from mothers was about the consistency of cooked vegetables and pulses about the raw ingredients used, and cooking methods for a particular food. The weight of chapattis, *paranthas*, etc., was also taken. The information of consumed cooked food was converted into raw equivalents. "The mean daily food intake was calculated by taking mean of three days intake and compared with Recommended Dietary Intake/Allowances by ICMR (Nutritive values of Indian foods by Gopalan et al. 2010)."

Food adequacy ratio (FAR) was calculated using the formula:

$$\text{FAR percent} = \frac{\text{Intake of foodstuff}}{\text{RDA}} \times 100$$

c) **Nutrient Intake:** Various nutrients, like energy, protein, fat, calcium, iron, and beta carotene was calculated using the food composition table (ICMR 2010 and https://ndb.nal.usda.gov/ndb/). The mean nutrient intake results

36

were compared with recommended dietary allowances for children (Nutritive values of Indian foods Gopalan et al. 2010). Nutrient Adequacy Ratio (N.A.R.) was calculated by using the following formula:

$$\text{N.A.R. \%} = \frac{\text{Intake of Nutrient}}{\text{RDA}} \times 100$$

Table 3.6 *Classification of N.A.R. %

Category	Range	Score
Adequacy	100 % & above	I
Marginally adequate	75-99.9%	II
Marginally inadequate	50-74.9%	III
Inadequate	Below 50%	IV

*Source Jood *et al.* 1999.

3.1.7 Preparation of education material and assessment of nutritional knowledge level:

A self-designed questionnaire assessed the nutrition knowledge, attitude, and practice of the mothers with 30 nutrition-based (food, nutrients, the role of healthy food, myths about nutrition, sources of nutrients, deficiency diseases, healthy cooking practices, etc.) questions. One mark given to correct answer, and zero marks given to incorrect answer. Total scores were recorded to reveal the extent of nutrition knowledge of the mothers. Score index of nutrition knowledge classified as follow:

Table: 3.7 *Nutritional Knowledge Score Index

Nutritional Knowledge Level	Scores
Very poor	0-5
Poor	6-10
Average	11-15
Good	16-20
Very good	21-25
Excellent	26-30

* Self-designed questionnaire

An education program through various approaches was framed for the mothers and children to impart awareness training. Multiple approaches were preferred by the researcher and organized programs for the children's benefits for their overall development in the studied area. The following program was organized:

1. Power point presentation.
2. Personal discussion with the mothers.
3. Display of charts and posters, and diagrams.
4. Leaflets and nutrition storytelling.
5. Nutritional videos.
6. Personal visits of some households.
7. An interaction and question-answer sessions.
8. Nutritional data through questionnaires:-   A- Knowledge

                                               B – Attitude

                                               C – Practice

1. **Power point presentation:** Power point presentation was carried out for the mothers to make them aware of the children's nutritional efficiency and deficiency and suggest necessary ways and means to the nutritional deficiency in the children. Side by side, specific valid questions were also answered.

2. **Display:** Various charts and diagrams were displayed at a centralized place, and necessary knowledge was compared to both mothers and children about nutrition issues and various economic sources of nutrition.

3. **Leaflets and nutrition story telling:** Necessary leaflets were distributed among mothers on the different issues related to prepare cheap nutritional food, certain stories about the effect of malnutrition on expectant mothers, lactating mothers, and children.

4. **Nutritional videos:** Videos containing important information and other aspects about nutrition in different states of the country, shown to the mothers to get knowledge about various types of food being consumed across the country by the children.

5. **Personal visits:** Most of the households were personally visited to see the environment where the food is being prepared, whether in hygienic conditions, the family members' eating habits were also noted.

6. **Interaction and questionnaires:** Many important questions raised by mothers/caregivers/grandparents were suitably answered for their benefits. They were pleased to know about certain nutritional aspects of various food items. Necessary information was delivered to the mothers for their day-to-day activities regarding food habits.

7. **Development of questionnaire regarding knowledge, attitude, and practice:** Wide discussion was held with the group of mothers of children under study regarding accepting the researcher's views regarding the nutritional issues prevailing in their respective areas. Accordingly, a questionnaire was developed (Annexure–2), which was further discussed with the senior faculty member's and peers groups. A few subject matter specialists were also consulted, and their views were also incorporated in the questionnaire. Ultimately a final shape was given by including all necessary information, knowledge, attitude, and practice.

Scoring Techniques:

a) **Knowledge Score:** The questionnaire contained 10 questions with four mutually exclusive alternatives and the correct one was given a score of one otherwise zero.

b) **Attitude :** The attitude scale were develop the 10 questions each having three alternative responses as:

    I.   **Strongly agree**

    II.   **Neither agree nor disagree**

    III.   **Strongly disagree**

These alternatives were score through a three-point likert's scale as follow:

    I.   **Strongly agree - 2**

    II.   **Neither agree nor disagree - 1**

    III.   **Strongly disagree - 0**

c) **Practice:** The practice scale was developed with ten questions having three alternative as :

These were quantified with the help of 3-point likert's scale as follow:

    I.   **Always- 2**

II.   Sometimes- 1

III.   Never- 0

IMPARTING NUTRITION EDUCATION

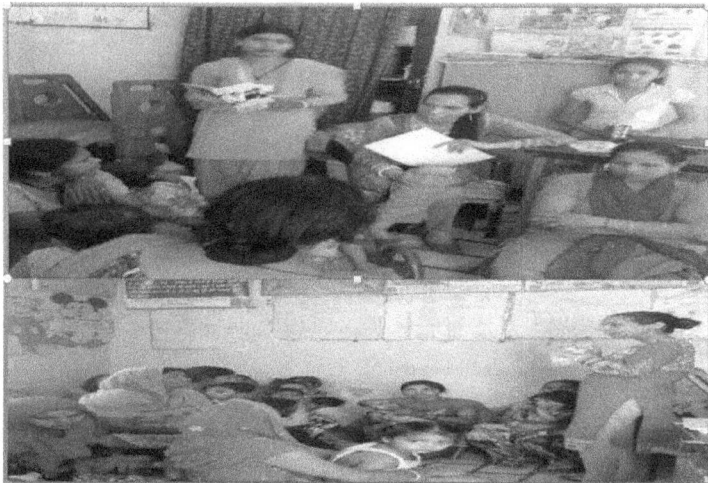

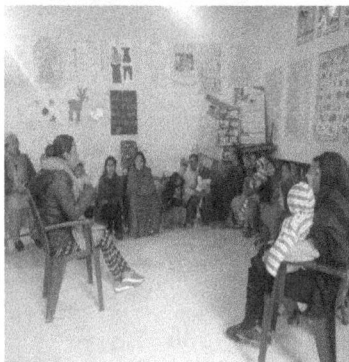

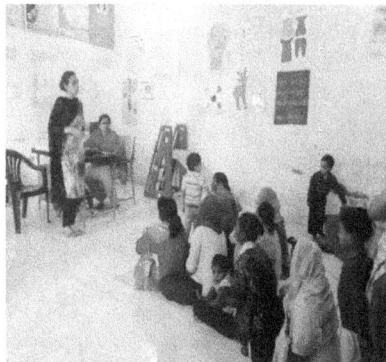

3.1.8 Development of enriched food preparations for nutrition interventions:

Value-added recipes like *Dalia*, *poshtik bhel*, and biscuits were developed by incorporating spirulina, roasted soybean, and soy flour, to improve energy's nutritional value, protein, fat, calcium, iron, and beta carotene. Organoleptic evaluation of the developed recipes was done in the department of home science using hedonic 9-point scale by ten judges comprising faculty members and research scholars, and the children's mothers.

Development of *Dalia* supplemented with spirulina

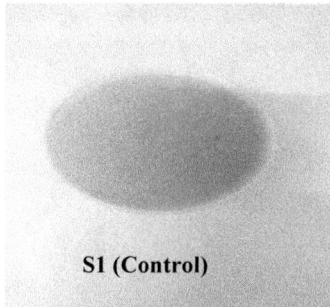
S1 (Control)

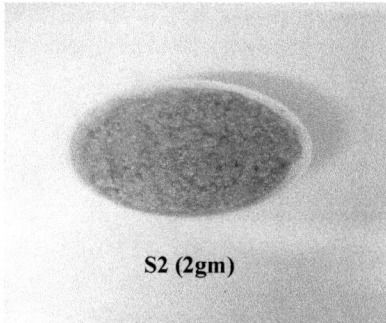
S2 (2gm)

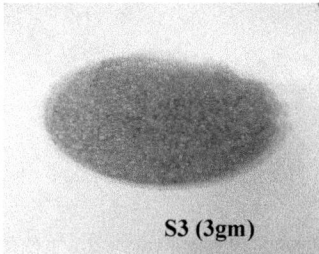
S3 (3gm)

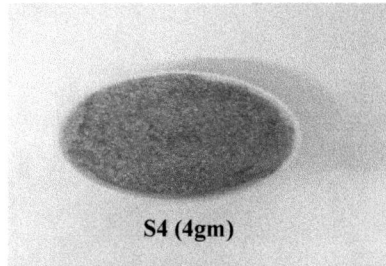
S4 (4gm)

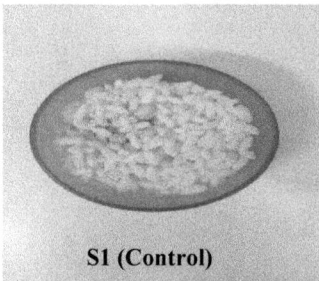
S1 (Control)

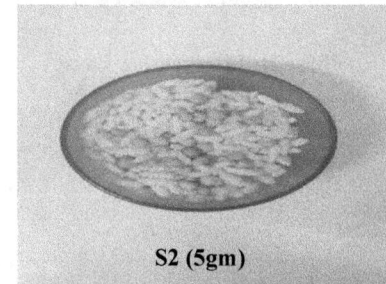
S2 (5gm)

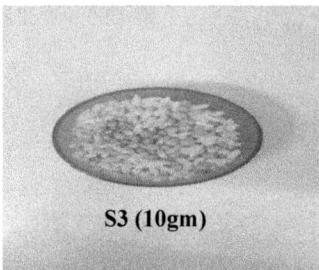
S3 (10gm)

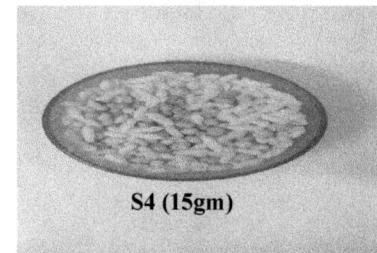
S4 (15gm)

Development of *Poshtik bhel* supplemented with roasted soybean

Development of Biscuits supplemented with soy flour

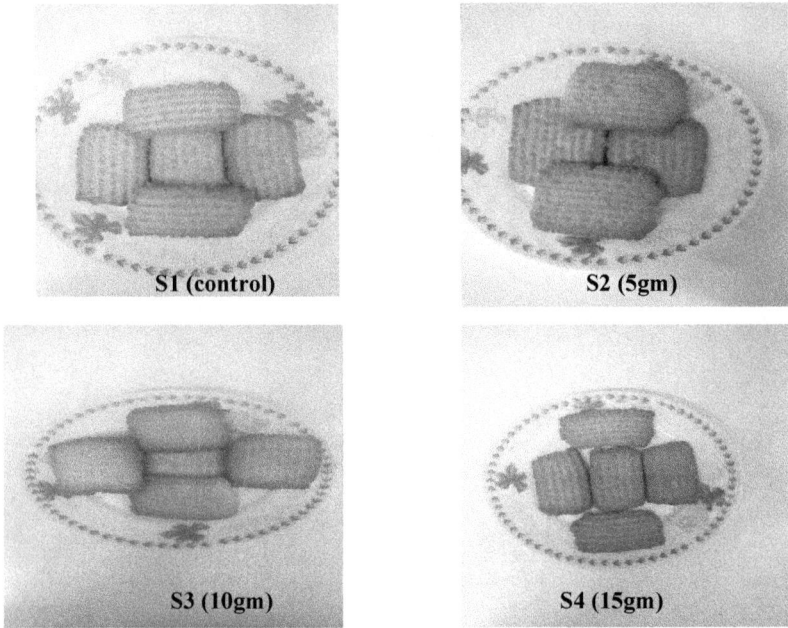

S1 (control)

S2 (5gm)

S3 (10gm)

S4 (15gm)

3.2   Phase II: Intervention Phase

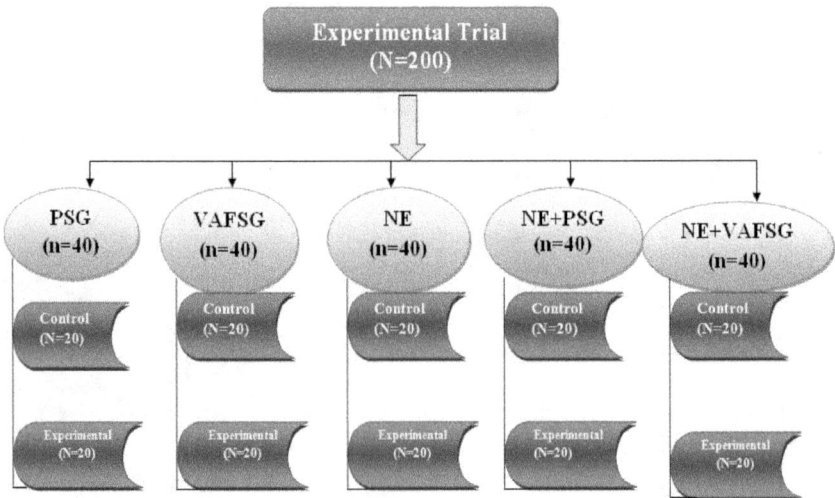

Fig.3.2 Experimental Plan

All the five groups which intervened with supplemented food combined up with control groups. Each intervention trial group and control group comprised 20 children. Out of the total number of children, 100 children aged 3-6 years preferred as the control group. The control group was not intervened with value-added food preparations, whereas 100 children were selected as the experimental subjects, which get involved with value-added recipes for the phase of four months.

Table: 3.8 Experimental Groups

Total children for feeding trials (n=100)				
Experimental Group I (n=20)	Experimental Group II (n=20)	Experimental Group III (n=20)	Experimental Group IV (n=20)	Experimental Group V (n=20)
Probiotic Supplemented group (PSG)	Probiotic supplemented + Nutrition education group (PSG+NE)	Nutrition Education group (N.E.)	Value-added food Supplemented group (VAFSG)	Value-added food supplemented group+ Nutrition education group (VAFSG+ NE)
Yakult	Yakult + N.E.	Imparted NE with various audio-visual aids	*Dalia, Poshtik-Bhel*, and Biscuits	*Dalia, Poshtik-Bhel*, Biscuits+NE

3.3 Phase III: Post-Intervention Phase

The impact of various nutrition interventions was assessed on anthropometric and biochemical parameters at 60 days i.e. mid of the study and after 120 days (after the complethion of interventions).

3.4 Statistical Analysis:

The data obtained all through the experiment trial was further diagrammatically tabulated and statistically analyzed to draw logical and scientific inferences. Most commonly used statistical test; mean, std. deviation, paired t-test, unpaired t-test, analysis of variance (ANOVA) and Tukey HSD test for multiple comparison.

CHAPTER - 4
RESULTS AND DISCUSSION

In the previous chapter 3, the planning of the experiment was discussed under the research methodology adopted. In this chapter (4), the execution part will be presented along with necessary information on various indicators, analysis and interpretation, and further discussion as per the study's objectives will be discussed.

4.1 General profile of pre-school children:

As per the sampling plan, two hundred pre-school undernourished children randomly selected from the study area were stratified into five strata. These strata of forty units, each with twenty control and twenty experimental, constituted the basis of the study.

Through the developed questionnaire, necessary data was collected from the purposively selected experimental children and their parents for their socio-economic profile (Table 4.1). The distribution of age suggested that the maximum (29.5%) children belonged to three years group followed by four (28%), five (22%) and six (20.5%) years. There were almost equal percentages of male (49.5%) and female (50.5%) children. Educational status showed that majority (68.5%) of the parents were illiterate; about 15 per cent of parents have acquired primary education, 14.5 percent were ended with metric and only 2 per cent have been over with intermediate. Most of the pre-school children parents belonged to labour class (58.5%) followed by servicemen (29.5%) and only 12 per cent were doing their own small business. Mothers of the maximum (53%) respondents were not working and about 47 per cent of the mothers were working. Nearly two-third (64%) of pre-school children belonged to nuclear family and one third (36%) had joint family. Annual income data of their family showed that for majority (59.5%), annual family income was between Rs.70000-1, 00,000, one fourth had more than a lakh and rest (15.5%) were having between Rs. 50000-70000 annualy. Maximum of the preschoolers were living in kutcha house (57.5%) followed by mixed (30%) and only 12.5 per cent were living in jhuggi.

Table-4.1 General Profile of the pre-school children

Variables		Frequency (n=200)	Percentage (%)
Age	3 Years	59	29.5
	4 Years	56	28
	5 Years	44	22
	6 Years	41	20.5
Gender	Male	99	49.5
	Female	101	50.5
Parental Education	Illiterate	137	68.5
	Primary Education	30	15
	Metric	29	14.5
Father Occupation	Intermediate	4	2
	Businessman	24	12
	Serviceman	59	29.5
	Labour	117	58.5
Mother Occupation	Working	94	47
	Not- Working	106	53
Family Type	Joint	72	36
	Nuclear	128	64
Income	50,000-70,000	31	15.5
	70,000-100,000	119	59.5
	More than lakh	50	25
House type	Katcha	115	57.5
	Mixed	60	30
	Jugghi	25	12.5

Fig. 4.1-4.4 Distribution of pre-school children according to general information

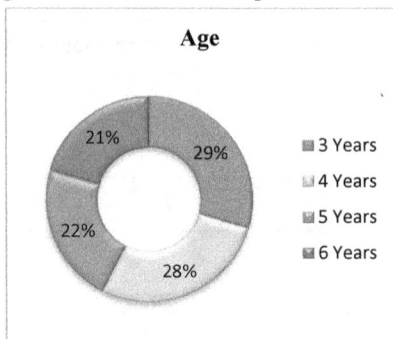

Fig.4.1

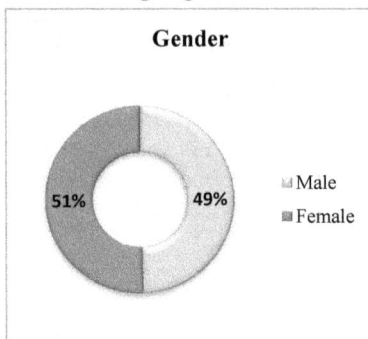

Fig.4.2

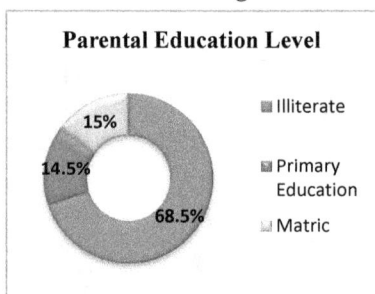

Fig.4.3

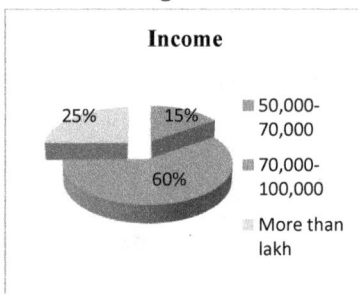

Fig.4.4

4.2 Clinical manifestation of pre-school children:

The clinical examination is further very important parameter for the assessment of nutritional level of the children. It was done to identify deficiency symptoms of various nutrients. The data pertaining to the clinical symptoms of the respondents has been presented in table 4.2. Lack of lustre in hair was observed amongst maximum (52%) pre-school children and dyspigmentation (18.5%) was also reported. Presence of pale conjunctiva was noticed in 40 per cent of the children; bitot's spot was also spotted but only in 3 per cent of the respondents; no children was identified with night blindness. It was pleasing to note that angular scars were found only in 14 per cent of the respondents and remaining (86%) were having normal lips. Maximum (80.5%) of the pre-school children had raw tongue. Mottled enamel and dental caries were more prominent only in 16.5 and 14.5 per cent children, respectively, which can be due to either of fluorine deficiency or bad brushing habits. Satisfyingly, most of the children had normal gums (88.5%), normal skin (87%) and normal nails (93%).

Table-4.2 Clinical manifestation among pre-school children

Variables		Frequency	Percentage (%)
Hair	Lack of lustre	104	52
	Dyspigmentation	37	18.5
	Normal hair	59	29.5
Eyes	Pale conjunctiva	80	40
	Bitot's spot	6	3
	Night blindness	0	0
	Normal eyes	114	57
Lips	Angular scars	28	14
	Normal pink lips	172	86
Tongue	Scarlet	11	5.5
	Raw tongue	161	80.5
	Normal tongue	28	14
Teeth	Mottled enamel	33	16.5
	Caries	29	14.5
	Normal teeth	138	23
Gums	Spongy gums	23	11.5
	Normal gums	177	88.5
Skin	Skin xerosis	0	0
	Pale	26	13
	Normal skin	174	87
Nails	Brittle nails	3	1.5
	Ridged nails	11	5.5
	Normal nails	186	93

4.5-4.8 Clinical manifestations (Hair, Eyes, Tongue and skin) among the pre-school children

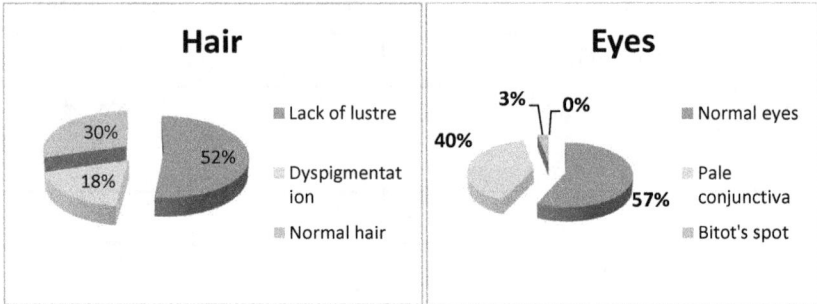

Fig.4.5   Fig.4.6

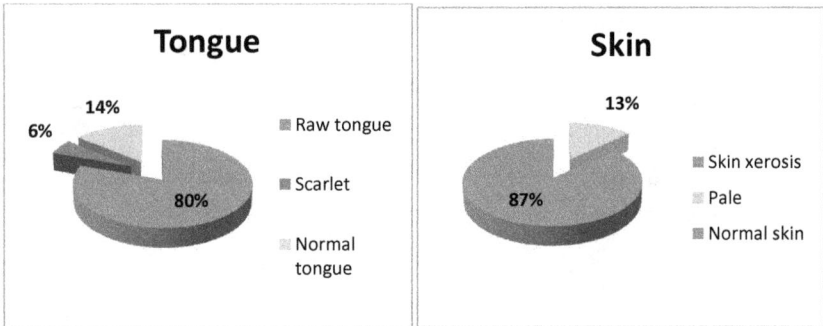

Fig.4.7   Fig.4.8

4.3 Dietary habits of pre-school children:

In response to classification on dietary habits as vegetarian and non-vegetarian, majority (97%) of the subjects were vegetarian and only 3 per cent were non-vegetarian. Out of non-vegetarians, chicken was preferred by maximum (83.33%) and only 16.66 per cent had liking for fish, however, non-vegetarian food was available hardly once a month to all (100%) of the subjects. Frequency of the meal intake responses revealed that majority (42%) of the respondents used to have two meals followed by once a day (30%) and only 28 per cent consumed three meals a day. Regarding skipping or missing the meal, response was 77.5 per cent affirmative and that too usually. The most skipped meal was breakfast (39.35%) followed by lunch (38.06) and evening meal (22.58). The reasons for skipping the meal were attributed as not tasty (19.35%), monotonous (14.19 %), no appetite (43.22%), and lack of time (23.22%). In response to nibbling, it was noticed that almost all (99.5%) nibbled;

48

maximum between lunch and dinner (65.82%), some in between breakfast and lunch (19.59%), also in dinner and bedtime (14.57%) if available. As far as snacks were concerned, almost 100 per cent loved snacking and street food. Most preferred snacks were chips (31.5%) followed by biscuits (28%), chocolates (21%) and crax (19.5%). While most liked street food preference wise were *chat/tikki* (25%), *samosa /bread pakora* (23.5%), hotdogs/ burgers (21.5%), *golgappa* (19%) and *bhelpuri* (11%).

Table-4.3 Dietary habits of pre-school children

n=200

Variables		Frequency (f)	Percentage (%)
Eating Habit	Vegetarian	194	97.0
	Non- Vegetarian	6	3.0
If Non-Vegetarian which Non-Veg. do you consume?	Chicken	5	83.33
	Fish	1	16.66
Frequency of consuming non-Veg.	Daily	0	0.0
	Once a week	0	0.0
	Twice a week	0	0.0
	Once in a month	6	100
Number of meals you consume in a day	One	60	30.0
	Two	84	42.0
	Three	56	28.0
Do you skip meal?	Yes	155	77.5
	No	45	22.5
If yes then	Usually	134	86.45
	Sometimes	21	13.54
Which meal do you skip most?	Breakfast	61	39.35
	Lunch	59	38.06
	Dinner	35	22.58

Reason of skipping meal	Not Tasty	30	19.35
	Monotonous	22	14.19
	Not Feeling Hungry/Cranky	67	43.22
	Lack of time	36	23.22
Do you nibble?	Yes	199	99.5
	No	1	0.5
If yes then what time?	In between breakfast and lunch	39	19.59
	In between lunch and dinner	132	65.82
	In between dinner and bed time	29	14.57
Do you like snacking?	Yes	200	100.0
	No	0	0.0
What do you prefer in snacking?	Biscuits	56	28.0
	Chips/Lays	63	31.5
	Kurkura/Crax	39	19.5
	Cookies/Chocolate	42	21.0
Do you like Street Food?	Yes	200	100.0
	No	0	0.0
If yes, then what do you like in junk food?	Hotdogs/Burger	43	21.5
	Bhelpuri	22	11.0
	Chat/Tikki	50	25.0
	Golgappa	38	19.0
	Samosa/Bread Pakoda	47	23.5

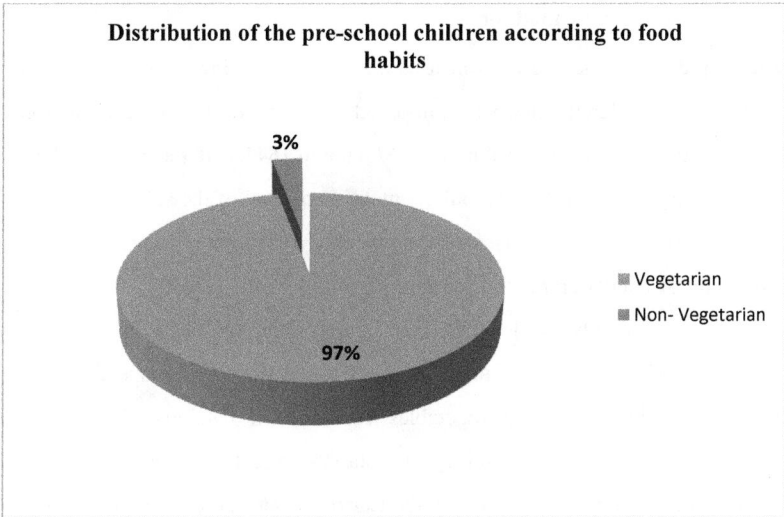

Distribution of the pre-school children according to food habits

3%

97%

- Vegetarian
- Non- Vegetarian

Fig.4.9

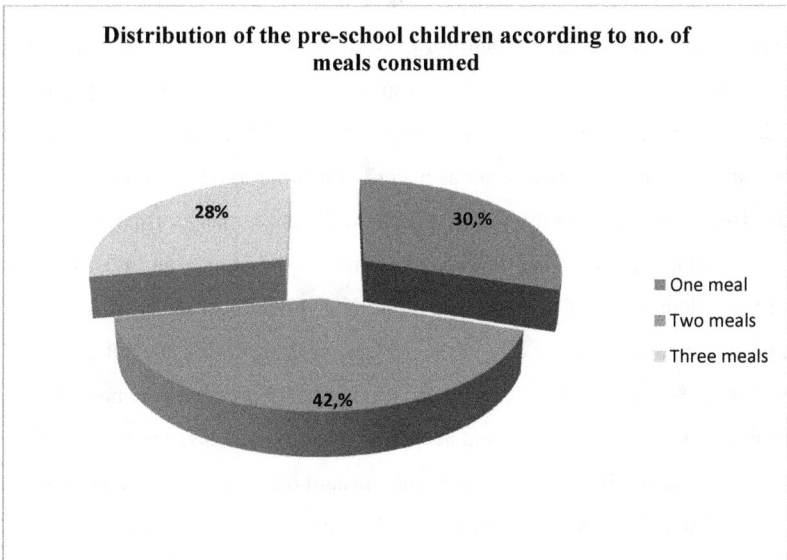

Distribution of the pre-school children according to no. of meals consumed

28%

30,%

42,%

- One meal
- Two meals
- Three meals

Fig.4.10

4.3.1 Frequency of daily food intake

The dietary data reported cereal wheat as a staple food being consumed on routine basis by all the children. Rice was consumed on alternate days (36.5) and weekly (54.5%) by the respondents (Table 4.4). Maximum (64%) of the children had not consumed maize extensively. The pulses intake frequency of the subjects had shown that the majority consumed pulses only on weekly and monthly basis. Frequency of consumption of bengal gram, and red gram by most of the subjects (53% and 44%) respectively was weekly, while black gram, green gram and *rajma* were consumed monthly. Vegetables are rich sources of roughage, β-carotene, iron and other vital vitamins and minerals. Leafy vegetables consumption data also indicated very deficient intake (monthly) for all the vegetables except for fenugreek which is reported to be consumed on weekly basis. Carrot, potato, onion and garlic were the main roots and tubers consumed daily by only 5, 62.5, 59.5, and 39.5 per cent of the respondents, respectively. Most (38.5%) respondents did not consume turnip, while tomatoes were consumed predominantly (78%) daily (as gravy/ *masala* preparations). Mainly beans, bitter gourd and cauliflower were consumed monthly, while peas were consumed weekly by 39 per cent of the respondents. Fruits (any) were not consumed on daily basis as fruits being pricey, might not reasonable by the families. The consumption of the fruits was fewer as majority (46%) of the children consumed only guava (seasonally) alternately, whereas fruits like banana, mango, papaya and jamun were consumed more either weekly or monthly depending on availability (as reported). More than half (52%) of the pre-school children consumed cow's milk on daily basis; almost equal per cent of the subjects consumed milk alternately (13.5%), weekly (15.5%) and monthly (15.5%) each and only 3.5 per cent were not in habit of consuming milk. Most of the subject never had curd, cottage cheese and buttermilk. In respect of fats and oil intake, vanaspati and mustard oil were consumed in routine by 45 per cent and 31 per cent respectively, while butter and *desi* ghee was not consumed by the majority. All the pre-school children had sugar intake on daily basis, whereas maximum (46.5%) of the respondents did not consume jaggery.

Table-4.4 Frequency of food groups intake among pre-school children

Variables	Food Stuffs	Daily	Alternately	Weekly	Monthly	Not consuming
Cereals	Wheat	200 (100)	0	0	0	0
	Rice	15 (7.5)	73 (36.5)	109 (54.5)	3 (1.5)	0
	Maize	6 (3)	39 (19.5)	18 (9)	9(4.5)	128 (64)
Pulses	Bengal gram	5 (2.5)	1 (0.5)	106 (53)	25 (12.5)	63(31.5)
	Black gram	0	17 (8.5)	70 (35)	93 (46.5)	20 (10)
	Green gram	0	52 (26)	51(25.5)	97 (48.5)	0
	Red gram	2 (1)	41 (20.5)	88 (44)	62 (31)	7 (3.5)
	Rajma	1 (0.5)	12 (6)	54 (27)	115 (57.5)	18 (9)
Leafy vegetables	Cabbage	0	15 (7.5)	43 (21.5)	108 (54)	34 (17)
	Spinach	0	29 (14.5)	71 (35.5)	98 (49)	2 (1)
	Feenugreek	0	21 (10.5)	91 (45.5)	74 (37)	14 (7)
	Mint	0	32 (16)	65 (32.5)	94 (47)	9 (4.5)
	Bathua	3 (1.5)	56 (28)	31 (15.5)	86 (43)	24 (12)
Roots and tubers	Carrot	10 (5)	85 (42.5)	43 (21.5)	62 (31)	0
	potato	125 (62.5)	75 (37.5)	0	0	0
	Onion	119 (59.5)	8 (4)	66 (33)	6 (3)	1 (0.5)
	Garlic	79 (39.5)	33 (16.5)	68 (34)	3 (1.5)	17 (8.5)
	Ginger	0	75(37.5)	73(36.5)	23(11.5)	29(14.5)
	Radish	0	95(47.5)	28(14)	59(29.5)	18(9)
	Turnip	0	47(23.5)	3(1.5)	73(36.5)	78(38.5)
Other vegetables	Tomato	156 (78)	44 (22)	0	0	0
	Brinjal	0	80 (40)	39 (19.5)	71 (35.5)	10 (5)
	Beans	0	4 (2)	45 (22.5)	139 (69.5)	12 (6)
	Bitter gourd	0	6 (3)	16 (8)	130 (65)	48 (24)
	Ridge gourd	0	62 (31)	20 (10)	42 (21)	26 (13)
	Bottle gourd	0	70 (35)	53 (26.5)	66 (33)	11 (5.5)
	Peas	0	40 (20)	78 (39)	76 (38)	6 (3)

	Cauliflower	0	13 (6.5)	52 (26)	127 (63.5)	8 (4)
Fruits	Guava	0	92 (46)	23 (11.5)	28 (14)	57 (28.5)
	Banana	0	33 (16.5)	17 (8.5)	25 (12.5)	125 (62.5)
	Orange	0	3 (1.5)	7 (3.5)	14 (7)	176 (88)
	Mango	0	43 (21.5)	24 (12)	40 (20)	93 (46.5)
	Papaya	0	33 (16.5)	34 (17)	43 (21.5)	90 (45)
	Apple	0	2 (1)	7 (3.5)	16 (8)	175 (87.5)
	Jamun	0	0	0	95 (47.5)	105 (52.5)
Milk & milk products	Cow's milk	104 (52)	27 (13.5)	31(15.5)	31 (15.5)	7 (3.5)
	Curd	8 (4)	14 (7)	25 (12.5)	42 (21)	111 (55.5)
	Cottage cheese	0	0	0	9 (4.5)	191 (95.5)
	Butter milk	0	0	26 (13)	29 (14.5)	145 (72.5)
Fats	Butter	0	0	11 (5.5)	10 (5)	179 (89.5)
	Desi ghee	0	2 (1)	3 (1.5)	4 (2)	191 (95.5)
	Vanaspati	91 (45.5)	31 (15.5)	1 (0.5)	2 (1)	75 (37.5)
	Mustard Oil	62 (31)	25 (12.5)	8 (4)	3 (1.5)	102 (51)
Sugar	Sugar	200 (100)	0	0	0	0
	Jaggery	8 (4)	70(35)	4 (2)	25(12.5)	93(46.5)

4.3.2 Mean daily food intake by the pre-school children

The study was carried out for estimation of daily food intake of the sample children under study. A sample of 200 was bifurcated into two as:

1) Control group (n=100)
2) Experimental group (n=100)

The mean daily food intake was analysed before (0day) and after (120days) experimental period separately for 3 years and 4-6 years age groups and the values were compared with RDA as specified in the table 4.5 for each age group. The response of each group i.e. 3 years and 4-6 years as revealed by the respondent's mothers regarding their food intake was recorded and results are summarizes in table.4.5

Table 4.5 Age-wise mean food daily intake of the pre-school children before and after imparting nutrition intervention

Food group (g/day)	RDA 1-3 yrs	Mean Daily Food Intake				Z Value				% change		t value	
		3 years (control n=24)		3 years (experiment n=35)		3 years (control)		3 years (After)		3 years (control)	3 years (experiment)	3 years (control)	3 years (experiment)
		Before	After	Before	After	Before	After	Before	After				
Cereal	60	20.75±3.26 (34.58)	20.18±2.61 (33.63)	19.81±1.89 (33.01)	21.56±1.92 (35.9)	-58.98	-74.74	-125	-118	-2.74	8.8	-1.00[NS]	-5.94**
Pulses	30	15.25±5.09 (50.83)	15.61±4.77 (52.03)	16.66±4.83 (55.53)	18.47±3.96 (61.56)	-14.19	-14.77	-16.33	-17.2	2.36	10.86	-2.02[NS]	-3.57**
Milk/milk products	500	42.62±11.38 (8.52)	41.37±13.23 (8.27)	34.28±13.37 (6.85)	39.52±11.49 (7.9)	-196.89	-169.8	-206.07	-237	-2.93	15.28	-1.88[NS]	-3.19**
Roots & tubers	50	20.18±2.63 (40.36)	19.86±2.24 (39.72)	19.95±1.73 (39.9)	20.76±2.33 (41.52)	-55.54	-65.91	-102.76	-74.2	-1.58	4.06	-2.16[NS]	-2.39**
GLV	50	21.37±3.08 (42.74)	21.37±3.08 (42.74)	18.80±1.59 (37.6)	19.81±2.17 (39.62)	-45.53	-45.53	-116.08	-82.3	0	5.37	-2.88**	-2.72*
Other vegetable	50	18.95±2.18 (37.9)	18.54±1.85 (37.08)	18.71±1.94 (37.42)	19.46±2.38 (38.92)	-69.77	-83.3	-95.41	-75.9	-2.16	4	-3.82**	-2.37*
Fruits	100	5.20±2.10 (5.2)	3.05±2.67 (3.05)	6.66±2.35 (6.66)	5.80±3.69 ((5.8)	-221.15	-177.9	-234.98	-151	-41.34	-12.9	1.62[NS]	2.22*
Sugar & jaggery	15	14.0±7.49 (93.33)	14.20±7.35 (94.66)	13.72±2.99 (91.4)	14.57±2.00 (97.1)	-0.64	-0.53	-2.53	-1.27	1.42	6.19	-3.94**	-2.20*
Fats and oil	25	9.37±2.18 (37.48)	9.58±2.15 (38.32)	6.85±2.13 (27.4)	6.90±1.94 (27.6)	-35.11	-35.13	-50.41	-55.2	2.24	0.72	-3.83**	-1.75[NS]

Food Groups	RDA(4-6 yrs)	Control n=76		Experimental n=65		Z Value				% change		t value	
Cereal	120	22.96±3.25 (19.13)	21.92±3.20 (18.26)	23.64±2.51 (19.7)	24.32±2.63 (20.26)	-260	-264.47	-309.5	-293	-4.52	2.87	4.13**	-3.24**
Pulses	30	21.38±4.36 (71.26)	21.34±3.93 (71.13)	21.92±4.06 (73.06)	21.56±3.69 (71.86)	-17	-19.21	-16.04	-18.4	-0.18	-1.64	.18[NS]	-2.03[NS]
Milk/milk products	500	37.99±10.32 (7.59)	38.83±12.43 (7.76)	41.94±13.27 (8.38)	45.64±9.89 (9.12)	-390	-323.44	-278.7	-370	2.21	8.82	-.68[NS]	-3.29**
Roots & tubers	100	22.80±3.52 (22.8)	22.14±3.24 (22.14)	23.12±2.86 (23.12)	24.05±3.20 (24.05)	-190	-221.09	-216.7	-191	-2.89	4	2.82*	-2.69*
GLV	50	22.98±2.92 (45.96)	22.35±3.24 (44.7)	23.8±3.79 (47.6)	24.55±3.26 (49.1)	-81	-74.39	-55.73	-62.9	-2.74	3.15	2.54*	-1.66[NS]
Other vegetable	100	20.43±2.69 (20.43)	19.97±2.68 (19.97)	21.25±2.93 (21.25)	23.41±3.09 (23.41)	-258	-260.33	-216.7	-200	-2.25	10.16	2.31*	-5.44**
Fruits	100	4.47±2.55 (4.47)	3.75±2.70 (3.75)	6.5±1.75 (6.5)	6.56±2.26 (6.56)	-327	-310.77	-430.6	-349	-16.1	0.92	3.36**	-.082[NS]
Sugar & jaggery	20	15.78±6.38 (78.9)	15.71±6.27 (78.55)	15.61±0.98 (78.05)	16.71±0.66 (83.55)	-5.8	-5.96	-1.14	-40.2	-0.44	7.04	.37[NS]	-7.50**
Fats and oil	25	10.37±2.60 (41.48)	10.46±2.68 (41.48)	9.53±2.15 (38.12)	10.15±2.56 (40.6)	-49	-47.29	-39.26	-46.8	0.86	6.5	-.61[NS]	-3.55**

Cereals: Mean daily intake of cereals by the preschoolers of experimental group (3years) was 19.81±1.89g/d and 21.56±1.92 g/d before and after the experiment period respectively. The results for 4-6 years age group subjects revealed that the daily average intake of cereals by pre-school children of experimental group was 23.64±2.51g/d and 24.32±2.63g/d before and after the nutrition intervention trial. Daily mean intake of cereals by the corresponding control subjects (before and after) of 3 years' and 4-6 years of age group were 20.75±3.26 g/d, 20.18±2.61g/d and 22.96±3.25g, 21.92±3.20g, respectively. An increment of 8.8 and 2.87 mean per cent change was observed in experimental group of both (3 and 4-6 years) the age group after the experimental trial. No improvement was found in the control group of 3 and 4-6 years age group at any stage of study trial. The results of z stastic (P≤0.01) of both (experimental and control) groups revealed the inadequate intake of cereals consumption among all the subjects as compared to RDA under study. Statistical analysis further reported that a highly significant improvement was in experimental group of both (3 and 4-6 years) age groups after four months of various intervention trials. On contrary results of control subjects of 4-6 years age group also showed significant (P≤0.01) difference at the end of the study. Study by Seid *et.al* (2018) is also in line with the findings of the study which revealed that 29 per cent of children were taking insufficient energy. The results of the present study are in agreement with the observation of Ghate (2014) who had also reported that the daily intake of cereals was deficient among the subjects.

Pulses: The mean daily pulse intake of experimental group of 3 years of age-group on before and after various nutrition interventions was 16.66±4.83g and 18.47±3.96gm respectively. For 4-6 years of age group the observed mean daily pulses intake by experimental respondents were 21.92±4.06g (before) and 21.56±3.69g (after) the experimental trial. The data (Table 4.5) revealed that the mean daily intake of pulses by the control subjects of 3 and 4-6 years age group (before and after) were almost similar i.e. 15.25±5.09, 15.61±4.77 and 21.38±4.36, 21.34±3.93. Maximum (10.86%) mean per cent change was observed in the experimental group of 3 years age-group. The Z values in respect of 3 years experimental and control subjects revealed a significant (P≤0.01) difference between RDA and actual consumption (before and after) of pulses intake. Further t stastic results revealed that highly significant ((p≤0.01) increment was found only in the experimental subjects of 3 years of age-group.

Milk and milk products: Mean daily intake of milk and milk products of experimental group (3 years) was 34.28±13.37 (before) and 39.52±11.49 (after). The percentage change was about 15.28 per cent. Average values of control group were 42.62±11.38 (before) and 41.37±13.23 (after). The mean percentage was almost of similar order. Through analysis, it was observed that the milk and milk product consumption for both the group before and after experimental period were quite deficient. This is also confirmed through t/z values (p≤0.01). From the data collected for 4-6 years age group, the average mean daily intake of milk and milk products by the subjects of experimental group was 41.94±13.27g and 45.64±9.89g before and after, respectively. Mean daily intake was lesser than the suggested RDA. The per cent change after experiment was about 8.82 per cent. Mean daily intake of milk and milk products for control group was 37.99±10.32g and 38.83±12.43g before and after trial respectively, with minor (2.21%) percentage change. The results in table 4.5 revealed that there is a great deficiency (P≤0.01) in intake of milk and milk products in the 4-6 years of age groups in comparison with RDA. This also needs to be suggested for correction to improve that level intake in sample children in the studied area. Statistical analysis revealed highly significant (p≤0.01) increment in the experimental group of both (3 and 4-6 years) the age category, while control group showed non-significant change. Dhanesh, (2016) also reported a significant improvement in consumption of all the food groups except milk and milk products among experimental group.

Roots and Tubers: Average daily intake of roots and tubers by 3 years of age group before and after 120 days of the experimental trial was 19.95±1.73g and 20.76±2.33g, with 4.06 per cent improvement. Respective mean values of control group were 20.18±2.63g (before) and 19.86±2.24g (after) with negligible percentage change. As per Z values significant difference between actual consumption and recommended dietary allowances was observed. Roots and tubers mean daily intake of 4-6 years of experimental children were 23.12±2.86g (before) and 24.05±3.20g (after) respectively. The percent intake was also low (23.12%) when compared with RDA. This is further confirmed through statistical analysis. The Z static is very high for all

58

the experimental indicators. The mean daily intake of roots and tubers by the respondents (4-6 years) of control group was almost of similar trend. There was non-significant change between both the stages (before and after).

Green leafy vegetable: Mean daily intake of green leafy vegetables by the experimental group (3years) before and after trial period was 18.80±1.59g and 19.81±2.17g. The percentage change was about 5.37 per cent at the end of the experiment. No change in mean intake of GLV was observed among control group. Although the consumption of green leafy vegetables is essential for growing children, the analysis suggested deficiency in consumption of green leafy vegetables in the entire control group. Statistically there exists a highly significant difference between RDA and actual availability ($p \leq 0.01$). The mean daily intake values before and after in respect of green leafy vegetables was 23.8±3.79g and 24.55±3.26g respectively in the experimental group of 4-6 years of age group. The data depicted in table 4.5 reported that the consumption of green leafy vegetables has a slight improvement in respect of per cent change before (0 day) and after (120days) trial period. Compared with RDA, all the indicators showed a significant difference between RDA and actual consumption by the sample children in the study area. The observed mean values of control group were of similar order. The results showed that mean percentage was declined after 120 days of experiment. Whereas t values of control group showed significant difference at 1 and 5 per cent in 3years and 4-6 years age group. However a significant ($p \leq 0.05$) change was also observed in experimental group of 3 years age group.

Other Vegetable: A miscellaneous group of vegetables was also considered for their availability to the respondents. The average values for 3 years of age group of the experimental group were 18.71±1.94g (before) and 19.46±2.38g (after), respectively. A slight (4%) per cent change was observed in the experimental group. Whereas the mean values of control group were 18.95±2.18g and 18.54±1.85 before and after. The availability of vegetables is almost of the same order but significantly different from RDA. The observed mean values before and after of 4-6 years of age group of the experimental group was 21.25±2.93g and 23.41±3.09 respectively. The result revealed an improved percentage change (10.16%) after the completion of the experiment. The revealed mean daily intake values of other vegetables of control group were 20.43±2.69g (before) and 19.97±2.68g (after) respectively. The decreased percentage change was observed between both (before and after) the stages. As summarized in table 4.5, the result confirms the deficiency in other vegetables intake also as the RDA is comparatively significantly higher (P≤0.01). The analysis further reported that there was significant difference at 1 per cent in the control group of 3 years and experimental group of 4-6 years. Whereas significant change at 5 per cent had shown in the experimental group of 3 years and control group of 4-6 years.

Fruits: Fruits are equally necessary for the growing children, but it is observed from the study that the availability of the fruit was almost zero-order compared to RDA. The observed mean intake of fruit in the 3 years of age group in the experimental group was 6.66±2.35g (before) and 5.80±3.69g (after). The negative values shown the deficient intake of fruit in the diet may be non-availability was the reason. The observed mean values before and after was 5.20±2.10g and 3.05±2.67g for control group. There was negligible percentage change. The mean values of fruit intake of experimental group for 4-6 years of the subjects were 6.5±1.75g and 6.56±2.26g before and after respectively, with negligible percentage change. The observed mean values of control group were 4.47±2.55g (before) and 3.75±2.70g (after). The percentage was declined at the end of experiment. The percentage for both the age group before and after showed a deficient intake of fruit in the diet. The intake of fruit by the subjects was deprived. A significant difference at 5 and 1 per cent in the experimental group of 3 years and control group of 4-6 years age respectively, was observed. A study conducted by Nolla et.al (2014) on the children (aged 0-5 years) of the rural area Bangang in Cameroon, also revealed low intake of fruit and vegetables. Sirasa et.al (2020) also reported inadequate amount of fruits and vegetables by the preschool children of urban region of Srilanka.

Sugar: The mean values of the experimental group (3 years) were 13.72±2.99g and 14.57±2.00g, respectively before and after the trial period. While the mean values of corresponding control group were 14.0±7.49g and 14.20±7.35g. The higher (6.19%) per cent change was observed as compared to control group (1.42%). There was no significant difference between consumption and RDA. The mean intake of sugar was also measured before and after in both the subgroup and compared with RDA for all the indicators. The before and after observed values (4-6 years) for both (control and experimental) the groups were 15.78±6.38g, 15.71±6.27g, and 15.61±0.98g 16.71±0.66g, respectively. There was increment in percentage (7.04) by the end of the experimental trial. The consumption of sugar and jaggery was sufficient when compared with recommended dietary allowances. Highly significant (p≤0.01) increment was found in the control group of 3 years of age and experimental group of 4-6 years group respectively.

Fat and Oil: The individual's consumption of fat and oil generally depends on all the family consumption. The mean values (3 years) depicted in the table before and after were 6.85±2.13g and 6.90±1.94g, respectively The percentage calculated revealed that there is deficient consumption of fat and oil per day. The average fat values of control group were 9.37±2.18g (before) and 9.58±2.15g (after). The percentage change was only about 2.24 per cent at the end of the experiment. However, the analysis suggested that the quantity consumed is significantly less (p≤0.01) than RDA. The result revealed that the daily mean intake of fats and oil of experimental group (4-6years) was 9.53±2.15g (before) and 10.15±2.56g (after) respectively. There was slight difference observed in percentage change as presented in table 4.5. A negligible change was reported for control group before and after the experiment. The insufficient intake of fat and oil was observed when compared to RDA. It was shown by the analysis may be attributed to the estimation method and a highly significant (p≤0.01) difference for all indicators. The analysis of t test revealed that highly significant (p≤0.01) difference was observed in the control group (3 years) and experimental group of 4-6 years age-group. Nasir *et.al* (2017) reported low fat consumption as compared to RDA by the children. Sati and Dahiya (2012) found in their study that the intake of pulses, cereals, green leafy vegetables, roots and tubers, other vegetables, milk and milk products, sugar and jaggery, fats and oil was significantly (p≤0.01) inadequate than the RDA. A similar study carried out on the children aged 1-6 years age group reported that intake of GLV (green leafy vegetable), fat, milk and milk products were lower than the RDA (Recommended dietary allowances (Chyne *et.al* 2017). Soni and Katoch ,(2014) also reported that the intake of all the nutrients except fat (significant at 5 per cent) was less than recommended allowances.

The result showed that the mean daily intake of food groups by the subjects was inadequate and lesser in both (before and after) the stages of control group when evaluated to suggested RDA. Whereas in the experimental trial group the consumption of food intake was also inadequate but the slight change was observed after the completion of experiment it can be concluded that different nutrition interventions can improve the dietary intake of the experimental sample.

Fig.4.11 Per cent intake of RDA of the pre-school children (3 Yrs)

Fig.4.11 Per cent intake of RDA of the pre-school children (3 Yrs)

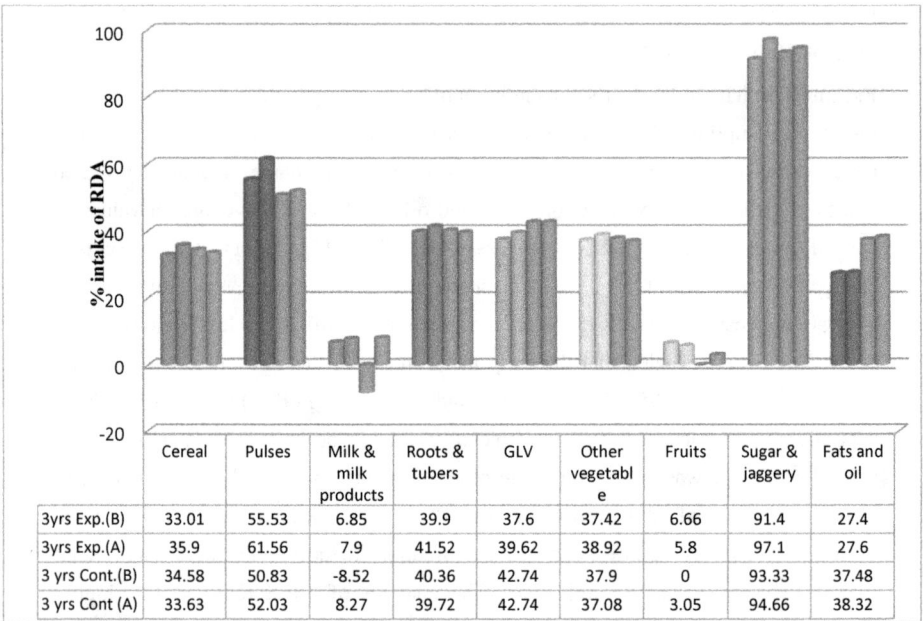

	Cereal	Pulses	Milk & milk products	Roots & tubers	GLV	Other vegetable	Fruits	Sugar & jaggery	Fats and oil
3yrs Exp.(B)	33.01	55.53	6.85	39.9	37.6	37.42	6.66	91.4	27.4
3yrs Exp.(A)	35.9	61.56	7.9	41.52	39.62	38.92	5.8	97.1	27.6
3 yrs Cont.(B)	34.58	50.83	-8.52	40.36	42.74	37.9	0	93.33	37.48
3 yrs Cont (A)	33.63	52.03	8.27	39.72	42.74	37.08	3.05	94.66	38.32

Fig.4.12 Per cent intake of RDA of the pre-school children (4-6 Yrs)

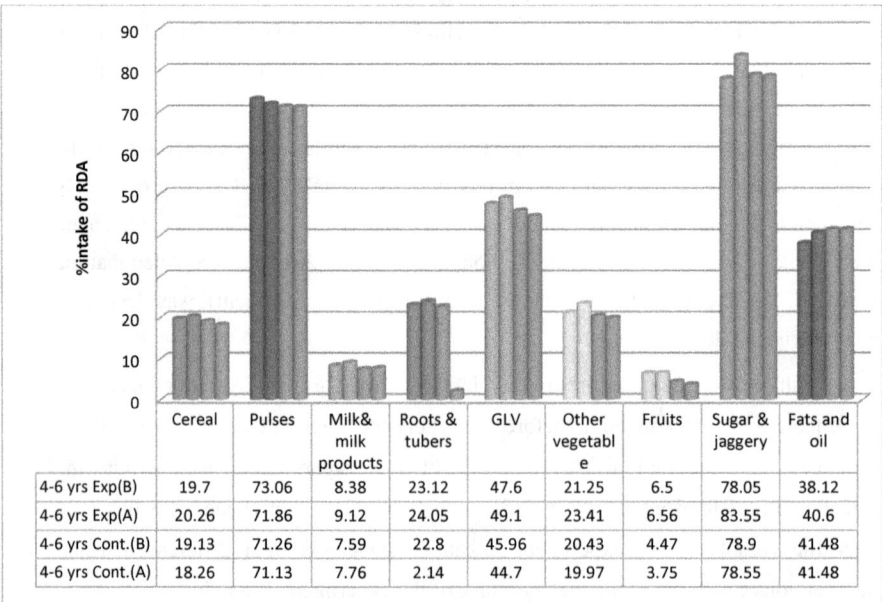

	Cereal	Pulses	Milk& milk products	Roots & tubers	GLV	Other vegetable	Fruits	Sugar & jaggery	Fats and oil
4-6 yrs Exp(B)	19.7	73.06	8.38	23.12	47.6	21.25	6.5	78.05	38.12
4-6 yrs Exp(A)	20.26	71.86	9.12	24.05	49.1	23.41	6.56	83.55	40.6
4-6 yrs Cont.(B)	19.13	71.26	7.59	22.8	45.96	20.43	4.47	78.9	41.48
4-6 yrs Cont.(A)	18.26	71.13	7.76	2.14	44.7	19.97	3.75	78.55	41.48

Fig. 4.13 Mean Percent change in food intake of pre-school children

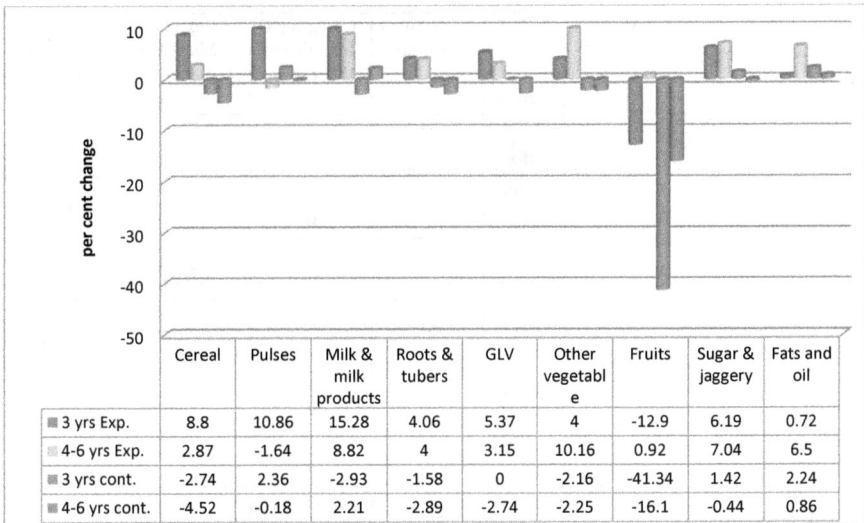

	Cereal	Pulses	Milk & milk products	Roots & tubers	GLV	Other vegetable	Fruits	Sugar & jaggery	Fats and oil
■ 3 yrs Exp.	8.8	10.86	15.28	4.06	5.37	4	-12.9	6.19	0.72
4-6 yrs Exp.	2.87	-1.64	8.82	4	3.15	10.16	0.92	7.04	6.5
■ 3 yrs cont.	-2.74	2.36	-2.93	-1.58	0	-2.16	-41.34	1.42	2.24
■ 4-6 yrs cont.	-4.52	-0.18	2.21	-2.89	-2.74	-2.25	-16.1	-0.44	0.86

4.3.2.1 Food adequacy ratio of daily food intake by pre-school children:

As discussed above in table 4.5, an attempt was made to analyze the daily food intake of different food groups in respect of the control group and experimental group. In order to discuss further the adequacy of the other group intake during pre and post-experiment under control and experimental group, a further stratification was done as follow:

1. Category I = 100% and above (Adequate)
2. Category II = 75% and above (Marginally adequate)
3. Category III = 50-74.9% (Marginally Inadequate)
4. Category IV = < 50% (Inadequate)

Adequacy of food intake (Experimental): The perusal of data showed that cereals, milk & milk products and fruits intake by all the subjects (before and after) were fell in the category IV (inadequate) No change was observed after intervention trial. 49 per cent of the respondents were having marginally inadequate amount of pulses before but it was 57 per cent (after) as decline of 3 per cent from inadequate category was observed. The decline of 1 per cent was seen in category II of pulses. Intake of roots and tubers was also for inadequate the subjects, however a slight improvement of 4 per cent was noticed from category IV (inadequate) to category II

63

Table 4.6 Food adequacy ratio of food intake by the pre-school children

Food Groups	Groups		Category I Adequate	Category II Marginally adequate	Category III Marginally Inadequate	Category IV Inadequate
Cereals	Experimental	Before	--	--	--	100
		After	--	--	--	100
	Control	Before	--	--	--	100
		After	--	--	--	100
Pulses	Experimental	Before	--	36	49	15
		After	1	36	57	6
	Control	Before	--	35	46	19
		After	--	34	50	16
Milk & milk products	Experimental	Before	--	--	--	100
		After	--	--	--	100
	Control	Before	--	--	--	100
		After	--	--	--	100
Roots & Tubers	Experimental	Before	--	--	--	100
		After	--	4	--	96
	Control	Before	--	--	1	99
		After	--	--	0	100
Green leafy vegetables	Experimental	Before	--	--	37	63
		After	--	--	38	62
	Control	Before	--	--	26	74
		After	--	--	27	73
Other vegetables	Experimental	Before	--	--	1	99
		After	--	--	1	99
	Control	Before	--	--	1	99
		After	--	--	--	100
Fruits	Experimental	Before	--	--	--	100
		After	--	--	--	100
	Control	Before	--	--	--	100
		After	--	--	--	100
Sugar	Experimental	Before	2	4	9	85
		After	2	7	9	82
	Control	Before	39	18	23	20
		After	38	20	25	17
Fats	Experimental	Before	--	--	3	97
		After	--	--	6	94
	Control	Before	--	--	14	86
		After	--	--	15	85

Figures in parenthesis are in percentage

(marginally adequate) after interventional trial except experimental subjects. and shifted to marginally adequate category. There was 1 per cent improvement for GLV. The percentage remained same before and after for other vegetables. Maximum of the preschoolers intake inadequate amount of sugar it remained same for category I and III. Whereas 3 per cent of the subjects moved from inadequate to marginally adequate category. The similar trend was found for fat where 3 per cent of the respondents shifted from category IV to III.

Adequacy of food intake (Control): It is revealed from the table (4.6) that sugar is the only food component that was intake in adequate amount in both the stages (before and after). It was found that pulses and sugar were falling in marginally adequate category but there was not much change was observed in both the stages of pulses and sugar. There was only 1 per cent change was seen in marginal adequate category of Root & tubers, GLV, other vegetables, sugar and fats respectively. The results concluded that intake of all the food components except pulses and sugar maximum of the respondents were in the inadequate category.

4.3.3 Mean daily nutrient intake by the pre-school children: The experiment was continued for four months to measure different daily nutrient intake, namely energy, protein, fat, iron, calcium, and beta-carotene in case of control and experimental groups. As in the previous experiment, the two age-specific groups, i.e., 3years and 4-6 years were analyzed statistically and discussed below:

Energy (kcal): Recommended Dietary Allowance (RDA) for energy intake for 1-3 years and 4-6 years age group are 1060 /day and 1350/day respectively. The results of present study divulged that the mean daily energy intake by the respondents of 3 years (experimental and control) before (0day) and after nutrition interventions trial period (120days) were 446.42±76.78kcal/d, 467.83±70.97kcal/d and 404.11±77.05 kcal/d, 397.53±73.61 kcal/d respectively (Table 4.7).The observed mean daily energy intake in 4-6 years age group (experimental and control) before and after were 489.95±75.40 kcal/d,505.73±72.65kcal/d and 518.15±93.22kcal/d, 510.6±87.05kcal/d respectively. The increased percentage changes among experimental subjects were 4.79 per cent and 3.22 per cent respectively, for 3 and 4-6 years age group after the experimental trial. Among control subjects a decline of -1.62 per cent in 3 years of age group and -1.45 per cent for 4-6 years age group, indicated further decreased intake of energy.

Table 4.7 Age-wise mean daily nutrients intake of pre-school children before and after imparting nutrition intervention

Nutrients	RDA 1-3 yrs	Mean Daily nutrient Intake				Z Value				% change		t value	
		3 years (control n=24)		3 years (experiment n=35)		3 years (control)		3 years (After)		3 years (control)	3 years (experiment)	3 years (control)	3 years (experiment)
		Before	After	Before	After	Before	After	Before	After				
Energy (kcal)	1060	404.11 ± 77.05 (38.12)	397.53±73.61 (37.50)	446.42 ± 76.78 (42.11)	467.83 ± 70.97 (44.13)	-42.27	-44.68	-47.9	-50.1	-1.62	4.79	2.20*	-3.08**
Protein (g)	16.7	14.27 ± 3.48 (85.44)	14.22 ± 3.77 (85.14)	9.48 ± 1.98 (56.76)	10.76 ± 2.03 (64.44)	-3.42	-8.15	-21.57	-17.31	-0.35	13.5	.065	-4.52**
Fat (g)	27	9.18 ± 3.06 (34)	9.17 ± 2.90 (33.96)	9.72 ±4.64 (34.33)	9.75 ± 4.03 (36.11)	-28.52	-30.12	-22.03	-25.32	-0.1	0.3	-.28	-.22
Iron (mg)	9	4.30 ± 1.10 (47.77)	4.02 ± 0.70 (46.66)	5.19 ± 0.97 (57.66)	5.97 ± 0.82 (66.33)	-20.93	-34.83	-23.23	-21.86	-6.51	15.02	.37	-3.03**
Calcium (g)	600	115.39 ± 25.66 (19.23)	116.66 ± 29.82 (19.44)	125.9 ± 22.09 (20.98)	134.92 ± 18.98 (22.48)	-92.52	-79.4	-126.96	-144.96	1.1	7.16	2.40	-3.92**
Beta carotene (µg)	3200	116.74 ± 61.05 (3.648)	128.58 ±53.24 (4.01)	269.55 ± 90.19 (8.42)	263.58 ± 69.37 (8.23)	-247.42	-282.62	-192.22	-250.42	10.14	-2.21	-1.06	.375

Nutrients	RDA 1-3 yrs	Mean Daily nutrient Intake				Z Value				% change		t value	
4-6 years Group		Control n=76		Experimental n=65									
		Before	After	Before	After	Before	After	Before	After				
Energy (Kcal)	1350	518.15 ± 93.22 (38.38)	510.6 ± 87.05 (37.82)	489.95 ± 75.40 (36.29)	505.73 ± 72.65 (37.46)	-91.96	-93.69	-77.79	-84.06	-1.45	3.22	1.31	-3.90**
Protein (g)	20.1	18.15 ± 4.02 (90.29)	17.66 ± 3.52 (87.86)	9.54 ± 2.25 (47.46)	10.80 ± 2.28 (53.73)	-37.83	-32.88	-1.07	-6.04	-2.69	13.2	1.76	-6.19**
Fat (g)	25	12.79 ± 4.60 (51.16)	12.63 ± 4.05 (50.52)	9.53 ± 3.34 (38.12)	10.08 ± 3.12 (40.32)	-37.34	-38.55	-23.14	-26.62	-1.25	5.77	1.22	-4.50**
Iron (mg)	13	4.40 ± 0.93 (33.84)	4.10 ± 0.68 (31.53)	5.03 ± 1.05 (38.69)	5.80 ± 1.0 (44.61)	-61.19	-58.04	-80.61	-114.1	-6.81	15.3	2.55	-2.74*
Calcium (mg)	600	161.80 ± 49.90 (26.96)	155.61± 45.45 (25.9)	133.69 ± 35.65 (22.28)	143.55± 27.04 (23.92)	-105.45	-136	-76.55	-85.33	-0.03	7.37	2.70	-6.103**
Beta carotene (µg)	3200	197.37 ± 59.94 (6.16)	190.94 ± 55.80 (5.96)	253.33 ± 131.97 (7.91)	278.86 ± 123.29 (8.71)	-180.01	-191.02	-436.7	-470.11	-3.25	10.07	1.72	-4.349**

**significant at p≤0.01, *significant at p≤ 0.05

66

A very high value of calculated Z static revealed significant ((P≤0.01)) difference between RDA and actual daily intake of energy among all the subjects of experimental and control groups at both the stages of trial period. Experimental subjects of both the age groups reported highly significant (P≤0.01) improvement for energy intake. On contrary, control subjects of 1-3 years age group showed significant decline regarding energy intake as compared to non significant intake for 4-6 years age group.

Protein: The observed daily protein intake of experimental group (3 and 4-6years) before and after nutrition interventions trial period were 9.48±1.98g/d, 10.76±2.03g/d and 9.54±2.25g/d and10.80±2.28g/d respectively as compared to recommended dietary allowances (RDA) of 16.7gm (3years) and 20.1gm (4-6 years) for protein. Mean daily intake of protein in the age group of 1-3 and 4-6 years control subjects (before and after) were 14.27±3.48g/d, 14.22±3.77g/d and 18.15±4.02g/d, 17.66±3.52g/d respectively.

An increment of mean per cent change of experimental group after 120 days of experimental trial was almost similar (13.2%-13.5%) for both the age groups. The mean percentage change in control group subjects showed decline of -0.35 and -2.69 per cent for both the age groups after studied period. Z static value of experimental group revealed that significant (P≤0.01) difference between RDA and actual intake of daily protein among all the subjects of experimental and control groups at both the stages of trial period. The analysis (t-value) further indicated that the experimental group showed highly significant (p≤0.01) improvement in intake of daily protein in the experimental sample children.

Fats: The mean daily fat intake by the respondents for 1-3 years (experimental and control) before (0day) commencing and after nutrition interventions trial period (120days) were 9.72±4.64g/d, 9.75±4.03g/d and 9.18±3.06 g/d, 9.17±2.09g/d respectively (Table 4.7). The observed mean daily energy intake in 4-6 years age group (experimental and control) before and after were 9.53±3.34 g/d, 10.08±3.12 g/d and 12.79±4.60 g/d, 12.63±4.05 g/d respectively. Negligible change was found in mean percentage (0.3%) change of experimental subjects of 3 years of age group. An

Fig. 4.14 Mean daily energy intake of pre-school children (3-6 years) before and after interventions

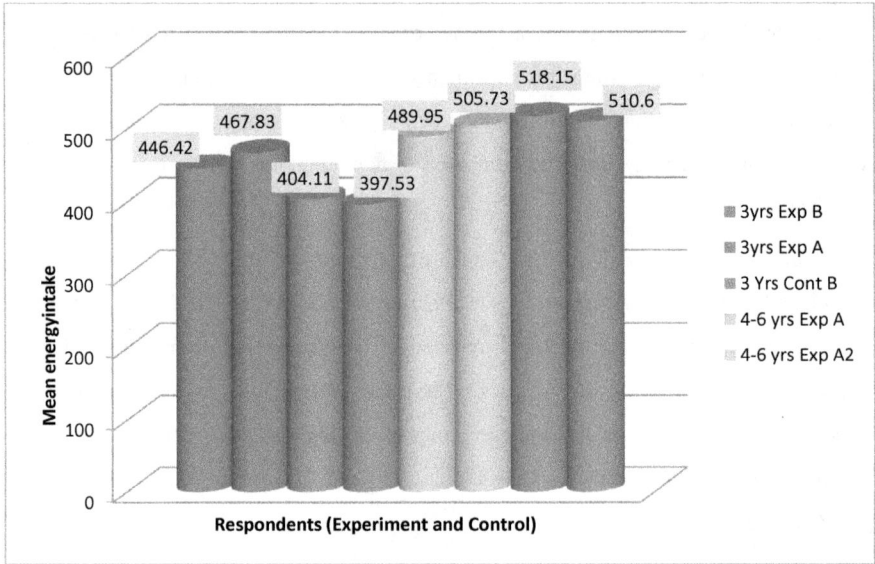

Fig.4.15 Per cent adequacy of energy intake of pre-school children (3-6 years)

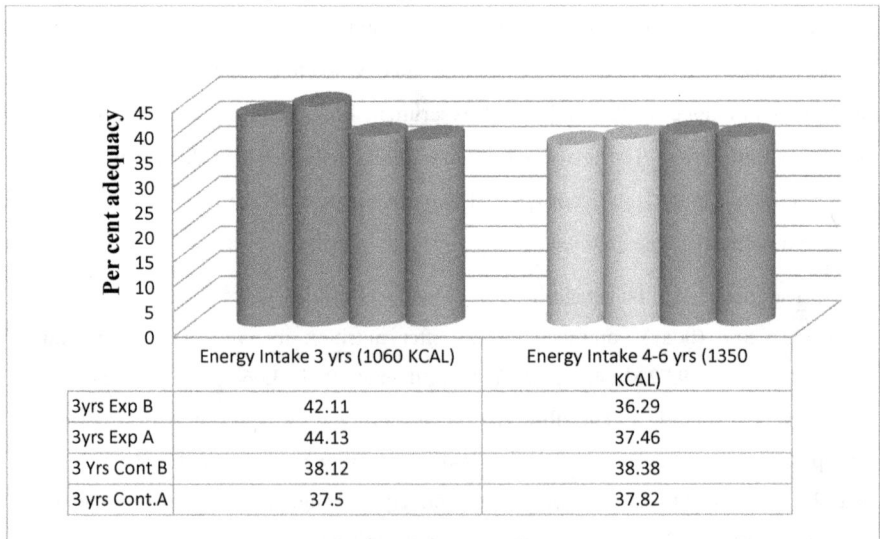

	Energy Intake 3 yrs (1060 KCAL)	Energy Intake 4-6 yrs (1350 KCAL)
3yrs Exp B	42.11	36.29
3yrs Exp A	44.13	37.46
3 Yrs Cont B	38.12	38.38
3 yrs Cont.A	37.5	37.82

Fig.4.16 Mean daily protein intake of pre-school children before and after interventions

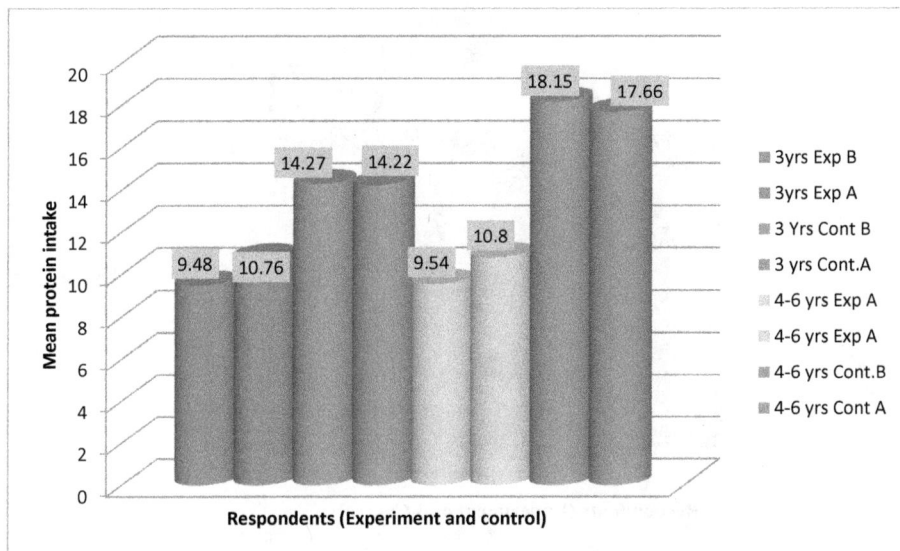

Legend:
- 3yrs Exp B
- 3yrs Exp A
- 3 Yrs Cont B
- 3 yrs Cont.A
- 4-6 yrs Exp A
- 4-6 yrs Exp A
- 4-6 yrs Cont.B
- 4-6 yrs Cont A

Values: 9.48, 10.76, 14.27, 14.22, 9.54, 10.8, 18.15, 17.66

X-axis: Respondents (Experiment and control)
Y-axis: Mean protein intake

Fig.4.17 Per cent adequacy of protein intake of pre-school children (3-6 years)

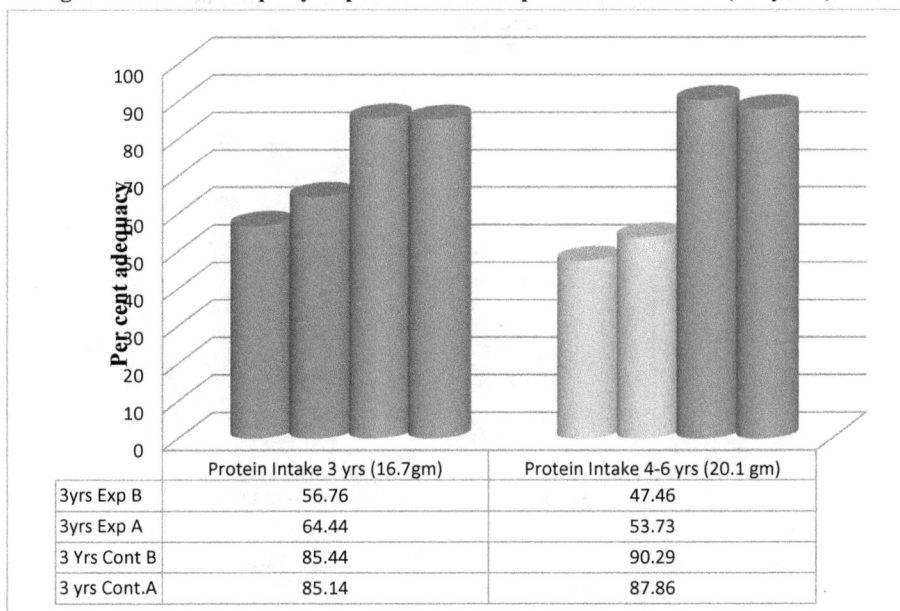

	Protein Intake 3 yrs (16.7gm)	Protein Intake 4-6 yrs (20.1 gm)
3yrs Exp B	56.76	47.46
3yrs Exp A	64.44	53.73
3 Yrs Cont B	85.44	90.29
3 yrs Cont.A	85.14	87.86

Y-axis: Per cent adequacy

Fig.4.18 Mean daily fat intake of pre-school children before and after interventions

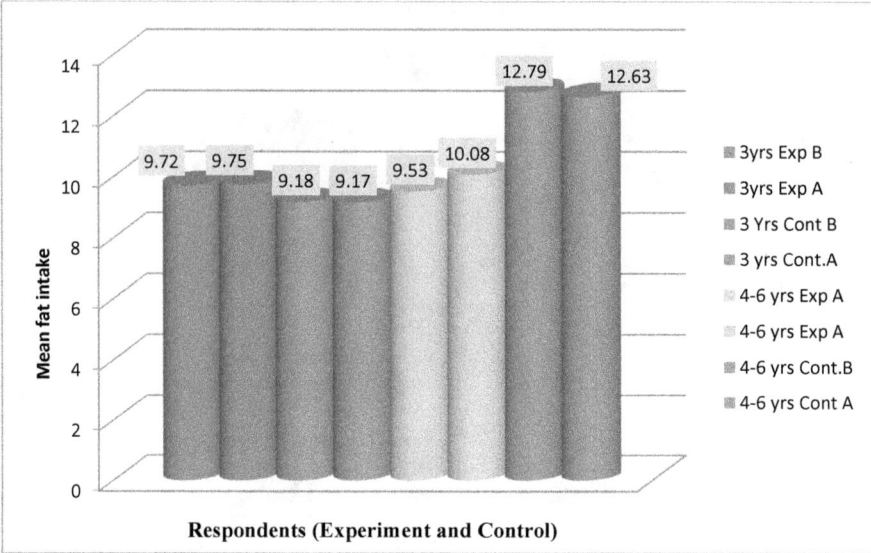

Fig.4.19 Per cent adequacy of fat in pre-school children (3-6 years) before and after interventions

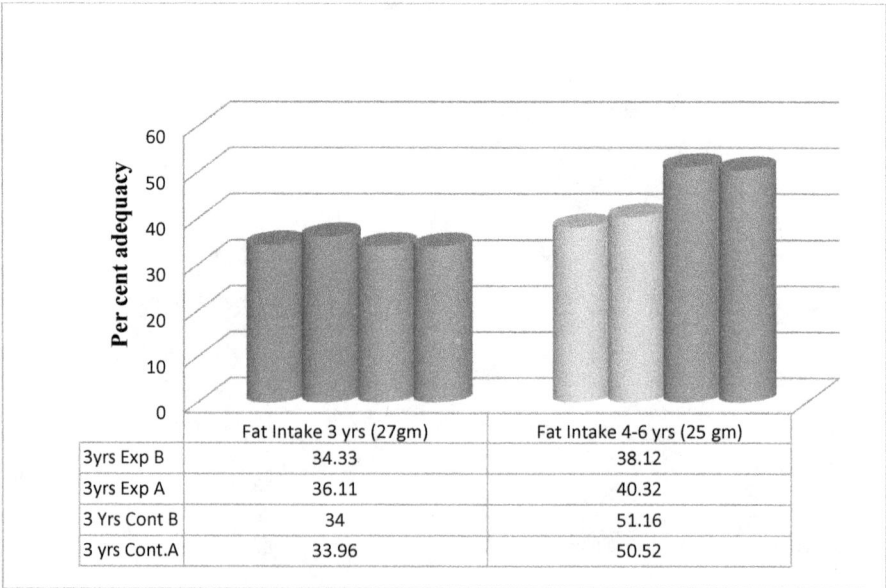

	Fat Intake 3 yrs (27gm)	Fat Intake 4-6 yrs (25 gm)
3yrs Exp B	34.33	38.12
3yrs Exp A	36.11	40.32
3 Yrs Cont B	34	51.16
3 yrs Cont.A	33.96	50.52

improved percentage change observed among experimental subjects of 4-6 years age group was 5.77 per cent after the completion (120days) of nutrition intervention trial (120days). Among control subjects a decline of -0.1 per cent in 3 years of age group and -1.25 per cent for 4-6 years age group, indicated further decreased intake of fat. A very high value of calculated Z static revealed significant (P≤0.01) difference between RDA and actual intake of fat among all the subjects of experimental and control groups at both the stages of trial period. Highly significant (P≤0.01) improvement for fat intake was observed only in 4-6 years age group after 120 days of experimental trial.

Iron: The mean iron intake by the subjects of experimental as well as control group in the age group of 3 years before and after were 5.19±0.97mg/d, 5.97±0.82mg/d and 4.30±1.10mg/d, 4.02±0.70mg/d respectively. In respect of 4-6 years of age-group mean iron intake by the respondents (experimental and control) before and after experimental trial were 5.03±1.05mg/d, 5.80±1.0 mg/d and 4.40±0.93 mg/d, 4.10±0.68 mg/d, respectively. The highest mean percentage was noticed (15.0 and 15.3%) in the experimental groups of both the age groups at the end (120days) of nutrition intervention trial. On contrary, control subjects of both the age group (1-3 and 4-6 years) showed decline mean per cent change regarding iron intake. A significant difference (P≤0.01) was observed between RDA and actual consumption of iron among all the respondents of experimental and control groups at both the stages of trial period. The results of t values revealed that highly significant (P≤0.01) improvement was observed in both the age groups (1-3 and 4-6 years) of experiment subjects after 120 days of nutrition intervention trial.

Calcium: Recommended dietary allowance of calcium (600mg) for 3 year age group is same as for 4-6 years. The average calcium intake per day by the respondents of experimental and control (3 and 4-6 years) before and after the experimental trial were 125.9±22.09mg/d, 134.92±18.98mg/d and 115.39±25.66mg/d, 116.66±29.82 mg/d respectively. For 4-6 years age group, the mean daily calcium intake of experimental as well as control group before and after were 133.69±35.65mg/d, 143.55±27.04mg/d and 161.80±49.90mg/d, 155.61±45.45mg/d respectively. The

Fig.4.20 Mean daily iron intake of pre-school children (3-6 years) before and after interventions

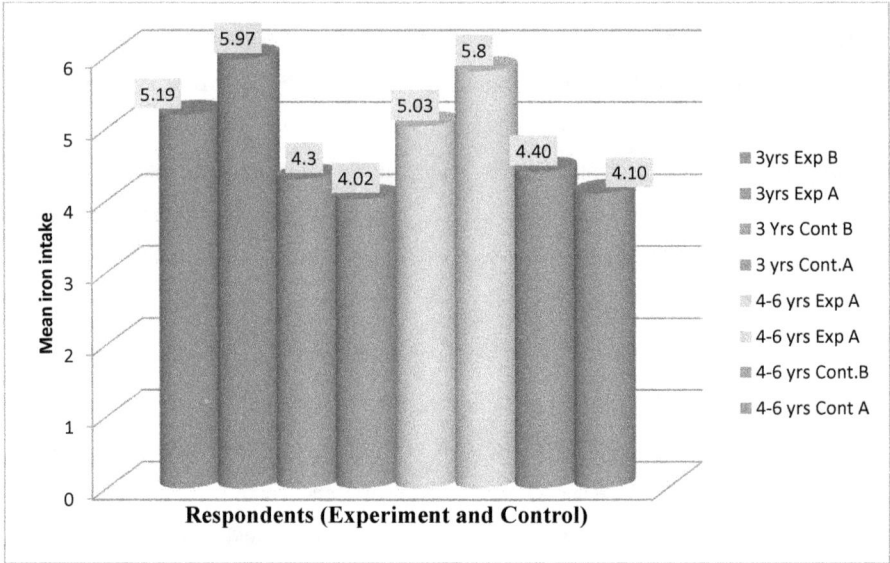

Fig.4.21 Per cent adequacy of iron intake of pre-school children (3-6 years) before and after interventions

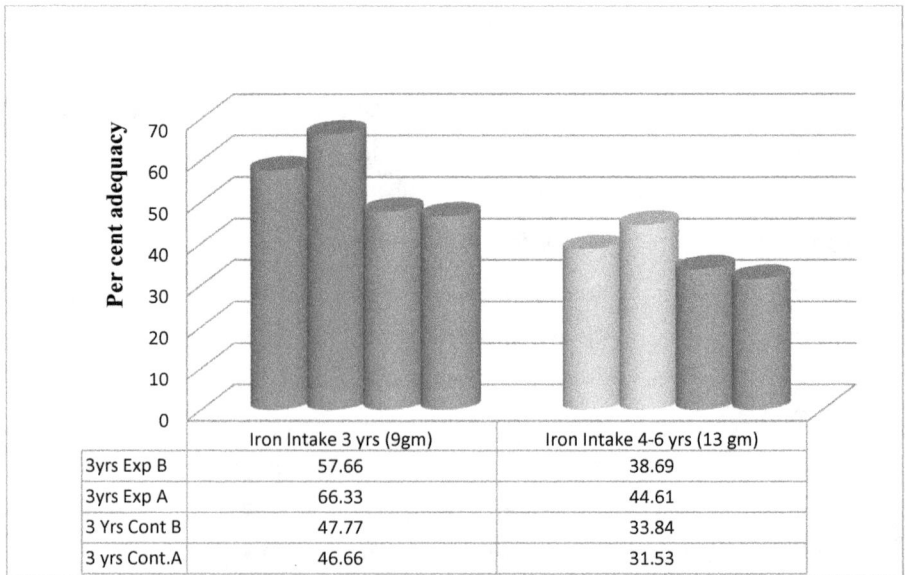

	Iron Intake 3 yrs (9gm)	Iron Intake 4-6 yrs (13 gm)
3yrs Exp B	57.66	38.69
3yrs Exp A	66.33	44.61
3 Yrs Cont B	47.77	33.84
3 yrs Cont.A	46.66	31.53

Fig.4.22   Mean daily calcium intake of pre-school children (3-6 years) before and after interventions

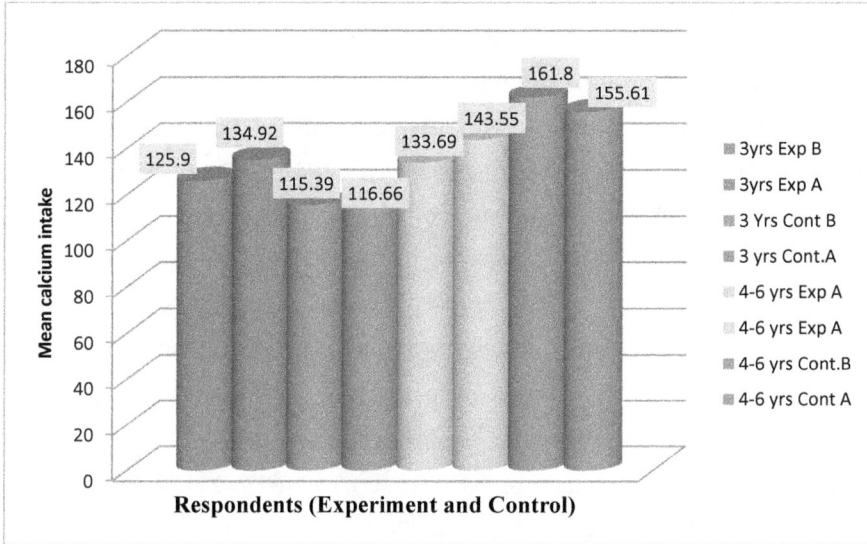

Fig.4.23 Per cent adequacy of calcium Intake of pre-school children (3-6 years)

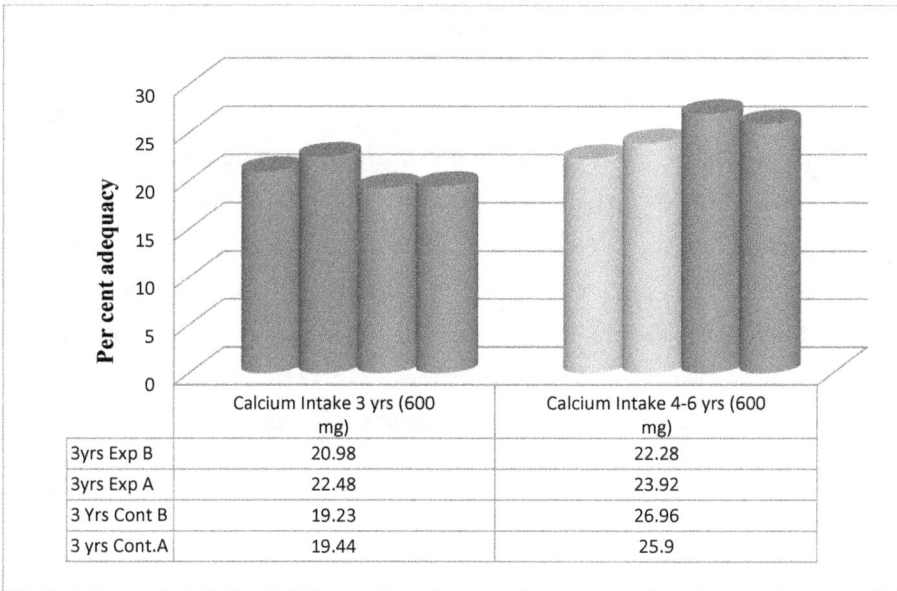

	Calcium Intake 3 yrs (600 mg)	Calcium Intake 4-6 yrs (600 mg)
3yrs Exp B	20.98	22.28
3yrs Exp A	22.48	23.92
3 Yrs Cont B	19.23	26.96
3 yrs Cont.A	19.44	25.9

mean per cent change of experimental group (before and after) completion of 120 days of nutrition intervention trial was almost similar (7.16% and 7.37%) for both the age groups. While, the percentage change is virtually negligible in the control group for both age groups (3 and 4-6 years) at the end of the study. Z static revealed that calcium content through various sources being consumed by the respondents was almost $1/4^{th}$ of the RDA in all the age groups at pre (0 day) and post-experimental (120 days) trial. Further statistical analysis of the data revealed a highly significant ($p \leq 0.01$) increment in calcium intake by the subjects (3 and 4-6 years) of experimental group after nutrition interventions trial. However, no significant improvement was observed in the control subjects after completion of study period.

β-carotene: The results of present study divulged that the mean daily β-carotene intake by the subjects of 3 years (experimental and control) before (0day) and after nutrition interventions trial period (120days) were 269.55±90.19μg/d, 263.58±69.37μg/d and 116.74±61.05μg /d, 128.58±53.24μg/d respectively (Table 4.7). The observed mean daily β-carotene intake in 4-6 years age group (experimental and control) before and after were 253.33±131.97μg/d, 278.56±123.29μg/d and 197.37±59.94μg/d, 190.94±55.80μg/d respectively. The increased percentage change among control subjects of 3 years age group was maximum (10.14%) after 120 days of study period. Almost similar per cent change (10.07%) was observed in experimental subjects of 4-6 years age group. A very high value of calculated Z static revealed significant ($P \leq 0.01$) difference between RDA and actual intake of β-carotene among all the subjects of experimental and control groups at both the stages of trial period. As per analysis in table 4.7 highly significant ($p \leq 0.01$) improvement was noticed only in the experimental respondents of 4-6 years age group at the end of the nutrition intervention trials. Study done by Navjot *et.al* (2016) is in line with present findings. They also reported inadequate intake of beta-carotene, energy, calcium and iron among preschool children of slum regions of Ludhiana

Fig.4.24 Mean daily β Carotene intake of pre-school children (3-6 years) before and after interventions

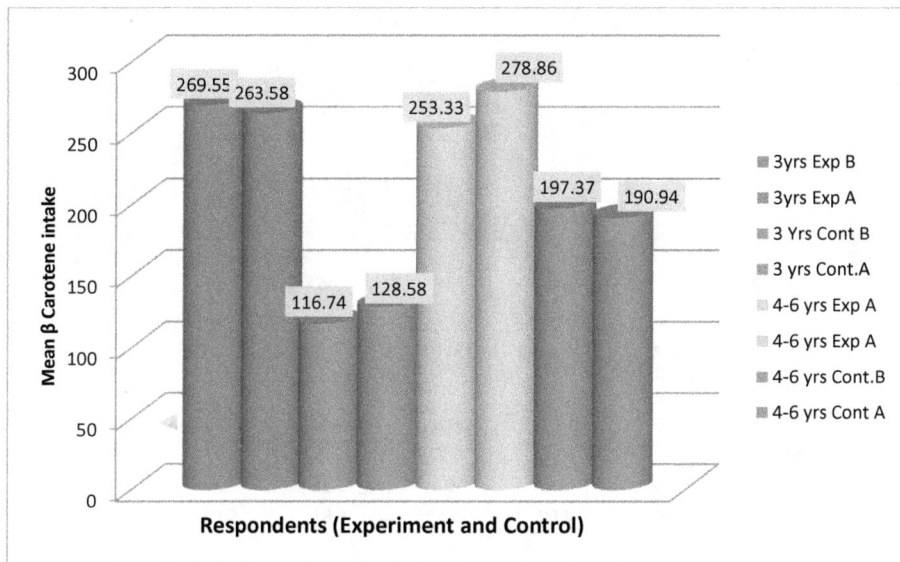

Fig.4.25 Per cent adequacy of β Carotene intake of pre-school children (3-6 years)

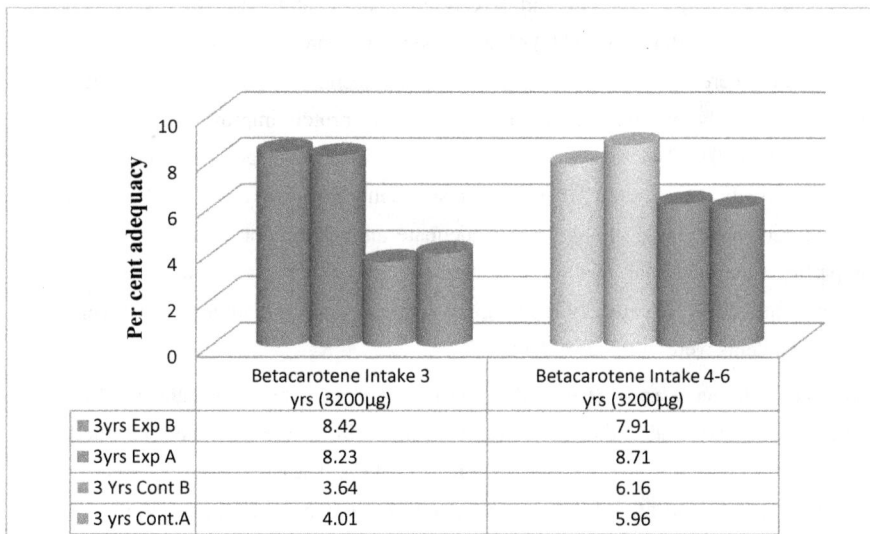

	Betacarotene Intake 3 yrs (3200μg)	Betacarotene Intake 4-6 yrs (3200μg)
3yrs Exp B	8.42	7.91
3yrs Exp A	8.23	8.71
3 Yrs Cont B	3.64	6.16
3 yrs Cont.A	4.01	5.96

Fig. 4.26 Per cent change in nutrient intake of pre-school children before and after nutrition interventions

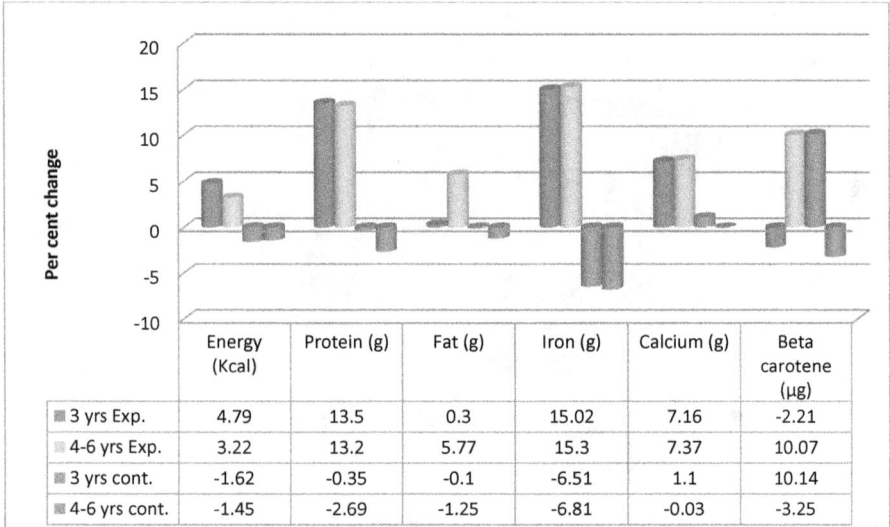

	Energy (Kcal)	Protein (g)	Fat (g)	Iron (g)	Calcium (g)	Beta carotene (μg)
3 yrs Exp.	4.79	13.5	0.3	15.02	7.16	-2.21
4-6 yrs Exp.	3.22	13.2	5.77	15.3	7.37	10.07
3 yrs cont.	-1.62	-0.35	-0.1	-6.51	1.1	10.14
4-6 yrs cont.	-1.45	-2.69	-1.25	-6.81	-0.03	-3.25

4.3.3.1 Nutrient adequacy ratio of food intake by the pre-school children

Nutrient adequacy ratio (Experimental): The data revealed that no change was observed for energy, calcium and β carotene before and after the experimental intervention. More than half (51%) of the respondents were having inadequate amount of protein, whereas 4 and 45 per cent of the respondents were in the category II and III respectively before the experiment. The intake of protein improved after 120 days of experiment. The 2 per cent of the respondents shifted to category III from category IV respectively. Maximum (71%) of the respondents iron intake was inadequate and 29 per cent were having marginally inadequate amount of iron in their diet before imparting interventional trial. The increment was found as 5 per cent of the respondents moved to category II (marginal adequate), whereas 46 and 49 per cent of the respondents were in category III and IV.

Nutrient adequacy ratio (Control): The observed percentage of category IV for control group concluded that there was no change in all the nutrients presented in table (4.8) before and after except protein (only 1%). The almost similar trend was observed before and after for category III except protein and iron (only 1%). The nominal percentage change was observed in protein due to some other reason or sampling error.

76

Table 4.8 Nutrient adequacy ratio of food intake by the pre-school children

Nutrients	Groups		Category I Adequate	Category II Marginally adequate	Category III Marginally Inadequate	Category IV Inadequate
Energy(kcal)	Experimental	Before	--	--	6	94
		After	--	--	6	94
	Control	Before	--	--	1	99
		After	--	--	1	99
Protein(g)	Experimental	Before	--	4	45	51
		After	--	10	37	53
	Control	Before	34	36	28	2
		After	30	43	26	1
Fat (g)	Experimental	Before	--	1	20	79
		After	--	1	22	77
	Control	Before	--	8	28	64
		After	--	7	29	64
Calcium (mg)	Experimental	Before	--	--	--	35
		After	--	--	--	35
	Control	Before	--	--	1	99
		After	--	--	1	99
Iron (mg)	Experimental	Before	--	--	29	71
		After	--	5	46	49
	Control	Before	--	--	14	86
		After	--	--	14	86
β carotene(μg)	Experimental	Before	--	--	--	100
		After	--	--	--	100
	Control	Before	--	--	--	100
		After	--	--	--	100

Figures in parenthesis are in percentage

Table 4.9 Sensory scores of organoleptic indicators of different value-added food preparations

Name of the recipes	Level of Incorporation	N	Color	Appearance	Aroma	Texture	Taste	Overall acceptability
Dalia	S1-(Control)	10	8.7±0.48	8.2±0.63	7.9±0.88	7.9±0.74	8.1±0.32	8.2±0.26
	S2-(1.7%=2gm)	10	6.8±0.79	6.8±1.23	7.5±0.97	7.9±0.74	8±0.47	7.4±0.41
	S3-(2.5%=3gm)	10	6.5±1.27	6.3±0.67	6.3±0.82	6.8±0.92	6.6±0.7	6.5±0.25
	S4-(3.4%=4gm)	10	6.3±0.95	6.3±1.64	6.4±0.7	6.6±0.97	6.3±0.95	6.4±0.5
	F		14.45**	6.39**	8.83**	6.79**	20.33**	50.2**
	CD (%)		1.12	1.37	1.03	1.03	0.79	0.45
Poshtik Bhel	S1-(Control)	10	7.4±0.84	7.6±0.7	7.5±0.97	8±0.82	8.6±0.7	7.8±0.66
	S2-(16.6%=5gm)	10	8.1±0.32	8.2±0.42	8.1±0.57	8.5±0.53	8.7±0.48	8.3±0.3
	S3-(33.3%=10gm)	10	6.9±0.57	7.1±0.32	6.8±0.79	6.7±1.06	6.4±0.84	6.8±0.46
	S4-(50%=15gm)	10	6.8±0.79	6.7±0.67	5.8±0.92	5.4±0.52	5.3±0.48	6±0.39
	F		8.05**	13.75**	14.29**	33.2**	28.16**	48.73**
	CD (%)		0.8	0.67	1	0.93	0.41	0.57
Biscuit	S1-(Control)	10	8.3±0.48	8.2±0.63	8.1±0.99	8.4±0.97	8.6±0.52	8.3±0.61
	S2-(25%=5gm)	10	8.8±0.42	8.7±0.48	8.7±0.48	9±0	9±0	8.8±0.23
	S3-(35%=10gm)	10	6.9±0.57	7.1±0.74	7.2±1.23	7.2±0.92	7.2±0.92	7.1±0.59
	S4-(40%=15gm)	10	7.3±0.67	7.2±1.03	6.9±1.29	6.8±1.32	6.3±1.64	6.9±1.01
	F		25.88**	10.81**	6.22**	11.96**	16.45**	19.54**
	CD (%)		0.66	0.91	1.29	1.14	1.18	0.81

Values are mean ± S.D ** Significant p≤0.01

78

4.4 Development of value-added food preparations

Dalia: *Dalia,* one of the wholesome food preparations, was prepared using standard recipe, i.e. (broken wheat and sugar) as control; to improve the nutritional value of *Dalia,* spirulina and peanuts were added as per following combinations:

a) S1 (CONTROL) : Broken Wheat (70gm), and sugar (30gm)
b) S2: CONTROL + 2gm (1.7%) spirulina and 5gm peanuts.
c) S3: CONTROL + 3gm (2.5%) spirulina and 5gm peanuts.
d) S4: CONTROL + 4gm (3.4 %) spirulina and 5gm peanuts.

Poshtik bhel: *Poshtik bhel,* as the name shows a nutritious snack prepared using puffed rice, roasted peanuts, and *channa* as control preparation. Roasted soybean was added in the following combinations to improve the nutritional value further:

a) S1 (CONTROL) : puffed rice (10gm), *channa* (10gm), and peanut (5gm)
b) S2: CONTROL + 5gm (16.6%) roasted soybean.
c) S3: CONTROL + 10gm (33.3%) roasted soybean.
d) S4: CONTROL + 15gm (50%) roasted soybean.

Biscuits: Biscuits are commonly prepared in many variations, and children are also fond of them. Therefore this product preparation was also tried in the present study with the following treatment combination:

a) S1 (CONTROL): Wheat flour (05gm), sugar (05gm), ghee (05gm), milk (2.5ml), and baking soda.
b) S2: CONTROL + 5gm (25%) of Soy flour.
c) S3: CONTROL + 10gm (35%) of Soy flour.
d) S4: CONTROL + 15gm (40%) of Soy flour.

4.4.1 Sensory evaluation: The value-added food preparations,like *Dalia, Poshtik bhel,* and Biscuits developed with different variations, were organoleptically acceptable. The acceptable level of supplementation varied in all the food preparation. However, mean sensory scores for all the characteristics declined on further supplementation beyond the accepted supplemented level.

DALIA: The mean score in respect of four variations under study, namely control (S1), *dalia* with 2gm (S2), 3gm (S3), and 4gm (S4) supplementation, are presented in table 4.9.

Colour: The most accepted supplemented level of spirulina was at 1.7 percent, as depicted by the highest mean colour score (6.8±0.79) among the three variants. The mean scores reduced (6.5±1.27) on increasing the per cent level of spirulina incorporation at 2.5 per cent, and at 3.4 per cent scores further decreased to 6.3±0.95. It is evident from the analysis that the F 14.45 was highly significant ($p \leq 0.01$), indicating no similarity between four groups of the recipe, including control. For further comparison of the mean scores, the critical difference at the 1% level was calculated. The difference between the control and all other groups was>1.12 in respect of *dalia* colour. Hence, it is concluded that the control group was significantly higher ($p \leq 0.01$) and different from the other three variations regarding color.

Appearance: The appearance of a product or preparation is equally important as that of color. The highest mean score of *dalia* regarding appearance was 8.2±0.63 in the control treatment. Mean scores decreased from 6.8±0.79 to 6.3±0.95 after the addition of spirulina at 1.7, 2.5, and 3.4 per cent as the colour of spirulina affects its appearance. A highly significant F statistic value (6.396) at a 1% significance level specified a significant difference between the four groups of *dalia* under study. A critical difference of 1.37 suggested that the control, i.e., S1 had a better appearance than the other three groups (S2, S3, and S4).

Aroma: S1 (control) scored the highest mean scores (7.9±0.88) for aroma among all the variants. On spirulina supplementation, maximum scores were gained by S2 (7.5±0.97) which, however, decreased to 6.4±0.7 (S3) and 6.3±0.82 (S4) on further increasing spirulina supplementation level. The analysis of the mean scores corresponding to aroma showed a significant difference (F 8.838 at $p \leq 0.01$) between four recipe groups. However, further analysis to compare the individual mean submitted that the control group (S1) and spirulina with 2gm (S2) did not differ and can be set to be of the same degree. Interestingly, the recipe containing 2gm of spirulina was significantly different ($p \leq 0.01$) from the other two groups. Hence, the addition of 2gm of spirulina (S2) can be accepted as a pleasing aroma and so also the control (S1).

Texture: The mean scores of *dalia* for texture revealed that the texture of both S1 and S2 were in a similar trend (7.9±0.74), whereas mean scores reduced at 2.5 per cent and 3.4 per cent (6.8±0.92and 6.6±0.97). The analysis revealed a highly significant difference (F statistics (6.791) at $p \leq 0.01$regarding texture. Further analysis suggested that S1 (control) and S2 (spirulina with 2gm) did not differ. However, S2 was significantly different from the other two groups, i.e., S3 and S4. Hence, the addition of 2gm of spirulina can be accepted as an excellent texture and control.

Fig.4.27 Mean overall sensory scores of value-added *Dalia.*

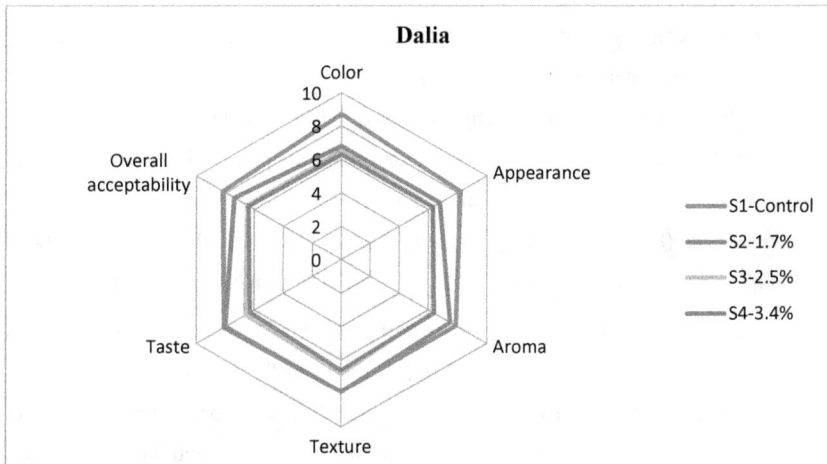

Taste: Taste is the prime factor associated with any product. Under sensory evaluation judgment on a 9- point hedonic scale, ten judges suggested that the mean scores vary from 6.3±0.95 to8.1±0.32 (table 4.9). The sensory mean scores for taste in S1 (control) and S2 *dalia* were very close, i.e., 8.1±0.32 and 8.0±0.47, whereas, on further addition of spirulina, the scores reduced to6.3±0.95. The analysis of variance suggested a very significant difference (F 20.338 at p≤0.01) among the four groups. The individual comparison of taste scores indicated that the critical difference (0.79) between S1 (control) and S2 (2gm of spirulina) was not similar. Similarly, a highly significant (p≤0.01) difference was noticed between S2 and the other two experimental groups of the recipe (S3 & S4).

Overall acceptability: Highly significant difference (F 50.2 at 0.455 CD) was observed statistically between all four variations of *dalia*. The sensory indicators suggested that *dalia* with 2gm of spirulina (S2) was quite acceptable for aroma, texture, taste, and overall acceptability among the three supplemented variations. Therefore organoleptically, S2 can be recommended for further use. The calculated value of F as 50.2 and CD .455 (p≤0.01) suggested a significant difference between the mean score; the control group was most acceptable, followed by 2gm, 3gm, and 4gm spirulina supplementation. Goel et al. 2011 also reported the acceptability of polyherbal mixture supplemented *dalia* at 2 percent.

Poshtik Bhel:

Colour: The mean score concerning colour was maximum (8.1±0.32) for S2, whereas the other three treatments (S1, S2, and S4) were awarded lesser scores 7.4±0.84 (S1), 6.9±0.57 (S3), and 6.8±0.79 (S4). The analysis of variance stated a highly significant difference (F 8.05, p≤0.01) between the four groups of preparations with a critical difference of 0.809. Further analysis specified that the preparation with 5gm of roasted soybean (8.1±0.32) was significantly different from the other two preparations (6.9±0.57, 6.8±0.79), but it does not differ significantly from control (7.4±0.84).

Appearance: In table 4.9, the mean scores of *Poshtik bhel* for appearance varied at different levels of supplementation. At 16.6 per cent of the incorporation of roasted soybean, appearance was best acceptable, i.e., 8.2±0.42, even better than the control sample (S1, 7.6±0.7). However, the rest two groups, S3 (33.3%) and S4 (50 per cent), showed decreased trends, i.e., 7.1±0.32 and 6.7±0.67. A highly significant (F value of 13.75) difference (p≤0.01) was observed regarding the appearance of *Poshtik bhel* in all the variations. Further analysis to compare individual mean with CD of .675 indicated a significant difference between S2 (5gm composition of roasted soybean) and all other supplemented variations. Therefore 5gm treatment (8.3±0.3) can be organoleptically recommended.

Aroma: The mean scores for aroma after addition of roasted soybean was highest at 16.6 per cent, while the control scored 7.5±0.97, and the other two treatments (S3 and S4) scored further lesser scores(6.8±0.79 for S3 and 5.8±0.92 for S4). It is evident from the table that the aroma effect was highly significant (F=14.29 p≤0.01andCD =1.009). A perusal of the data specified that the mean difference with 5gm roasted soybean treatment (8.1±0.57) was comparatively higher than the other two treatment groups (6.8±0.79, 5.8±0.92), suggesting a significant difference. Still, it was not so with control (7.5±0.97). However, the control was significantly different, respectively, with 10gm and 15gm composition. The highest value of mean sensory scores as 8.1±0.57 was fairly sufficient to conclude that the developed food preparation (*Poshtik bhel*) at 16.6 per cent was satisfactorily accepted for aroma.

Fig. 4.28 Mean overall sensory scores of value-added *Poshtik bhel*

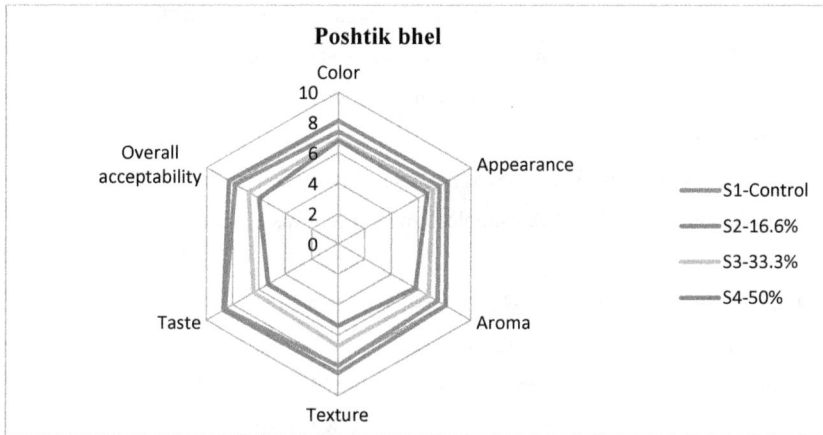

Texture: The mean scores for texture presented in table 4.9 showed that S2 scored maximum at 16.6 per cent level of supplementation. On further supplementation of roasted soybean at 33.3 per cent and 50 per cent the mean scores reduced to 6.4± 0.84 (S3) and 5.4±0.52 (S4). A highly significant F statistic (33.27) in respect of texture indicated a significant difference (p≤0.01). Further comparison with critical difference CD=.932 specified that the addition of 5gm roasted soybean (8.5±0.53) differs significantly with 10gm (6.7±1.06) and 15gm (5.4±0.52), respectively. However, the mean scores of S1 (control) and S2 (5gm) were non-significant. Because of the highest mean organoleptic scores (8.3±0.3), there is no reason to reject 5gm roasted soybean (8.7±0.48) composition for texture also.

Taste: The initial taste score (S1) observed was 8.6±0.7, while the taste of the S2 treatment was most acceptable and awarded with a score of 8.7±0.48. However, after the addition of roasted soybean at 33.3 per cent and 50 per cent the mean scores were reduced to 6.4±0.84 (S3) and 5.3±0.48 (S4). F=67.60, a critical difference of .788, is summarized in table 4.9. The individual comparison of the mean score for taste suggested that S1 (control) and S2 (5gm soybean addition) were almost on the same wavelength but differed significantly (F=67.60 and a critical difference of .788) with the other two preparations, i.e., S3 (10gm) and S4 (15gm). It is evident from the table 4.6 that control (without supplementation) and 5gm roasted soybean supplementation both were equally effective in respect of taste which can be safely accepted.

Overall acceptability: The best overall acceptability mean score was 8.3±0.3 at 16.6 per cent of supplementation. The analysis showed a significant difference (p≤0.01) between all the four variants of *Poshtik bhel*. The overall acceptability of *Poshtik bhel* based on mean scores suggested the treatment group 5gm scored maximum followed by control, 10gm, and 15gm roasted soybean variant. Statistical analysis also suggested (F value= 48.73, CD=.575, p≤0.01) a significant difference between mean scores. The 5gm roasted soybean supplemented group was most acceptable.

Biscuits:

Colour: The scores for colour characteristics after adding soy flour in the biscuits varied from 6.9±0.57 to 8.8±0.42. The study showed that supplementation of soy flour in the wheat flour at different levels, i.e., 10, 15, 20, and 25 per cent for value-addition, scored for the sensory attribute as 6.9 to 8.1, respectively (Murlidhar2016). The mean scores, as detailed in table 4.9 were further tested for the significance of the difference using ANOVA. The calculated value of F=25.88 was found to be highly significant (p≤0.01), and the critical difference of 0.0665 suggested that S2 (preparation with 5gm of soy flour addition) was significantly higher than the other preparations, namely S3 and S4 respectively, with 10gm & 15gm of soy flour supplemented food preparations. However, its comparison with the control group didn't show any significant difference, but the control group had a comparatively lower mean score. A perusal of the data recommended that the treatment group with 5gm of soy flour addition was reasonably satisfactory regarding colour attribute.

Fig. 4.29 Mean overall sensory scores of value-added Biscuits

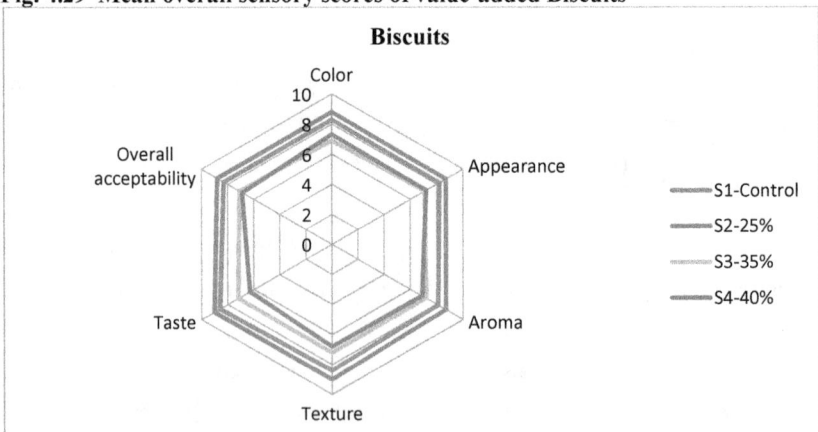

Appearance: The mean appearance scores in biscuits were found maximum for S2 treatment, i.e., 8.7±0.48. S1 as control (no value addition) scored 8.2±0.63. S3 and S4 scored almost identical mean scores, i.e., 7.1±0.74 and 7.2±1.03. Sensory evaluation scores analysis reported the highest appearance mean scores (8.7±0.48) for 5gm soy flour addition. The pattern of mean scores as per table 4.8 was similar to that of the colour as discussed above. Analysis of variance observed the F-value as 10.81(p≤0.01) with CD=9.14 depicted significant difference.

Aroma: After incorporating soy flour in the biscuits, the mean scores for S2 treatment was 8.7±0.48, whereas control (S1) scored 8.1±0.99. Decreasing scoring trend was noticed after including soy flour further beyond the acceptable level (S3, 7.2±01.23 and S4 6.9±1.29). Organoleptically, S2, i.e., value addition with 5gm soya flour, received the highest mean score (8.7±0.48), followed by S1 (control, 8.1±0.99), S3 (7.2±1.23 in 10gm soy flour), and S4 (6.9±1.29 in 15gm soy flour) (table 4.9). The aroma mean scores also showed a similar trend as that of color and appearance. ANOVA suggested (F value of 6.22 with CD 1.299 highly significant (p≤0.01) difference among the variants as compared to the S2 variant.

Texture and Taste: Texture and taste are the two most vital characteristics of any food preparation. The judge's evaluation scores indicated almost a similar trend for these two sensory attributes, as shown in Table 4.9. The most appropriate scores for texture and taste were at a 25 per cent level of supplementation, i.e.9.0±0. However, respective fewer scores were awarded to the other two treatments (S3 and S4) after value addition, i.e., 7.2±0.92, 6.8±1.32 (texture) and 7.2±0.92, 6.3±1.64 (taste). The analysis of variance (table 4.9) suggested a calculated value of F as 11.96 with CD 1.144 (p≤0.01) and 16.5 with CD 1.188 (p≤0.01); a highly significant difference (p≤0.01) between mean scores of texture and taste, respectively. No significant difference between S1 and S2 was noticed. However, a significant difference was observed between S2and S3 & S4 variations each. Sensory analysis for texture and taste attributes opened full scores (out of 9) for the treatment S2 (combination with 5gm soy flour). Hence it is concluded that the biscuit prepared with the addition of 5gm soy flour was better acceptable.

Overall acceptability: The overall acceptability for the treatment group with 5gm (25%) soy flour addition was found to be the most acceptable, followed by control, 10

85

gm soy flour, and 15 gm soy flour. The analysis of variance suggested a highly significant difference between mean scores among the variants. The present study's findings are in line with the outcomes of Tasnim Farzana and Suman Mohajan (2015). They showed that biscuits with soy flour substitution, up to 20 per cent were nutritionally superior to the whole wheat flour biscuits. Goel and Kaur (2013) also described the acceptability of polyherbal mixture added biscuits. TJ Kaur (2009) and T. Kaur and M.sharma (2015) developed and assessed the organoleptic acceptability of value-added local food preparations for combating malnutrition. Godson 2014 also favoured the sensory evaluation of the food preparations for assessing the acceptability of the improved recipe. Therefore, sensory evaluation is very much recommended for evaluating the community acceptability of value-added local food preparations that can be used to improve the nutritional status, hence combating malnutrition.

4.5 Efficacy of nutrition interventions on nutritional status of pre-school children

Each nutrition intervention group was further divided into control and experimental subgroups with 20 undernourished pre-school children each. The measurement were based on the system of experimentation as before (0day), during (60days), and after (120days) levels and further statistically analysis to draw logical and scientific inferences. Mean scores, mean change and t value (paired t test) has been also presented in the respective tables of the parameters under study. The mean changes were taken corresponding to B/D, D/A, and B/A respectively (in per cent). Since the subjects under study were taken as the dependent samples for B/D/A the paired t test was the most appropriate to compare the effects.

4.5.1 Efficacy of nutrition interventions on Height of the pre-school children

Height of the experiment as well as control sub-group samples was measured corresponding to nutrition interventions, namely PSG, VAFSG, NE, NE+PSG, and NE+VAFSG as per standard method using a vertical scale. The statistical analysis of the data so generated on height has been presented in table 4.10.

PSG: The mean height values of the probiotic supplemented experiment and control sub-groups were 89.95±5.04 cm, 89.95±5.04 cm, 90.40±4.97cm and 91.85±3.95cm, 91.85±3.95cm 92±41.10 cm at starting (0day), after 2 months (60days) and after 4 months (120days) of the trial period. Per cent change in height (0.5%) for experimental sub-group was three times more as compared to control sub-group

Table: 4.10 Efficacy of nutrition interventions on the Height of the pre-school children during different stages of interventions

Nutrition Interventions		Actual Increase			Mean change						t value		
		Before (0day)	During (60days)	After (120days)	B/D (0-60days)		D/A (60-120days)		B/A (0-120 days)		B/D (0-60days)	D/A (60-120days)	B/A (0-120days)
					Total	%	Total	%	Total	%			
PSG	Control	91.85±3.95	91.85±3.95	92±41.10	0	0	0.15	0.2	0.15	0.2	0.000	1.831	1.831
	Experimental	89.95±5.04	89.95±5.04	90.40±4.97	0	0	0.45	0.5	0.45	0.5	0	3.943**	3.943**
VAFSG	Control	88.50±1.96	88.55±1.90	88.75±1.91	0.05	0.1	0.2	0.2	0.25	0.3	1	2.179*	2.517*
	Experimental	87.15±4.09	87.15±4.09	87.65±3.99	0	0	0.5	0.6	0.5	0.6	0	3.68**	3.68**
NE	Control	88.85±4.09	89.95±4.08	90.10±4.03	0.1	0.1	0.15	0.2	0.25	0.3	1.453	1.831	2.517**
	Experimental	90.10±4.12	90.10±4.12	90.20±4.09	0	0	0.1	0.1	0.1	0.1	0	1.453	1.453
NE+PSG	Control	89.25±3.66	89.40±3.67	89.80±3.87	0.15	0.2	0.4	0.4	0.55	0.6	1.83	3.559**	4.06**
	Experimental	92.10±6.41	92.25±6.55	92.25±6.55	0.15	0.2	0	0	0.15	0.2	1.83	0	1.83
NE+VAFSG	Control	89.15±2.64	89.15±2.64	89.20±2.64	0	0	0.05	0.1	0.05	0.1	0	1	1
	Experimental	88.45±3.31	88.60±3.36	89.40±3.26	0.15	0.2	0.8	0.9	0.95	1.1	1.83	5.14**	6.19**

**significant at p≤0.01, *significant at p≤ 0.05

CONTROL– No Intervention

PSG- Probiotic supplemented group; VAFSG –Value-added food supplemented group; NE –Nutrition education; NE+PSG- Nutrition education+ Probiotic supplemented group; NE +VAFSG – Nutrition education + value -added food supplemented group

B/D – Before / During D/A- During/ After B/A– Before/ After

(0.2%). Growth in height was statistically significant (p≤0.01) after 2 months (0-60days) and 4 months (0-120days) of probiotic feeding. The findings by Kong *et.al,* (2021) showed that probiotic significantly improved height of the subjects in experiment trial group as compared to control group

VAFSG: The experimental sub-group subject's mean height values were 87.15±4.09cm, 87.15±4.09cm and 87.65±3.99cm whereas control sub-group's were 88.50±1.96 cm, 88.55±1.90 cm and 88.75±1.91cm before (0day), during (60days) and after (120days) the studied period, respectively. Experimental sub-group subjects supplemented with value added food preparations has shown good expected effects (0.6% improvement) with significant (p≤0.01) change for D/A (60-120days) and B/A (0-120days).The mean per cent change was not so high (0.3%) for the control sub-group, but t statistics have shown a significant difference (p≤0.05) for D/A (60-120days) and B/A (0-120days) after nutrition interventions trial. Since the control group has been not given any nutrition intervention, the changes in D/A (60-120days), B/A (0-120days) may be attributed to natural change subject to sampling fluctuation.

Fig.4.30 Mean Height of pre-school children during different stages of nutrition interventions

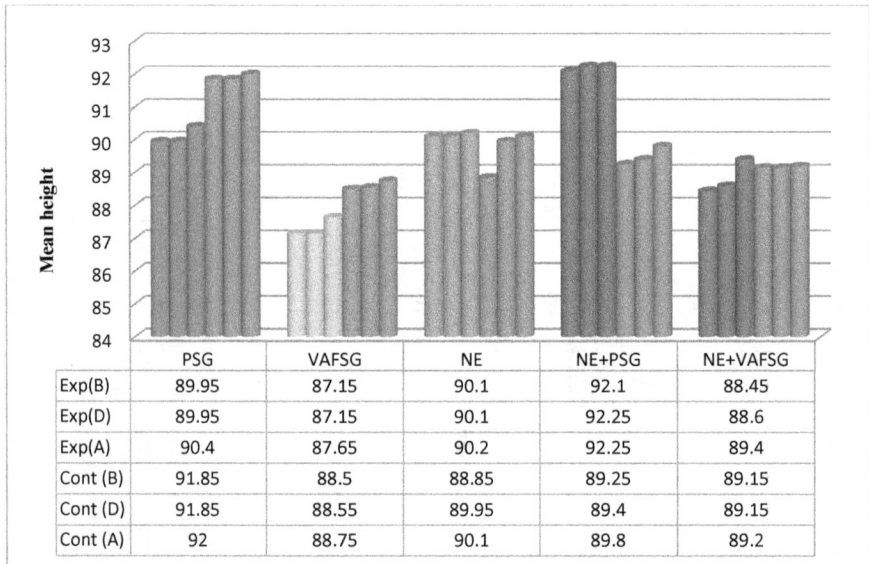

	PSG	VAFSG	NE	NE+PSG	NE+VAFSG
Exp(B)	89.95	87.15	90.1	92.1	88.45
Exp(D)	89.95	87.15	90.1	92.25	88.6
Exp(A)	90.4	87.65	90.2	92.25	89.4
Cont (B)	91.85	88.5	88.85	89.25	89.15
Cont (D)	91.85	88.55	89.95	89.4	89.15
Cont (A)	92	88.75	90.1	89.8	89.2

Fig.4.31 Per cent change in Height of the pre-school children before during and after intervention

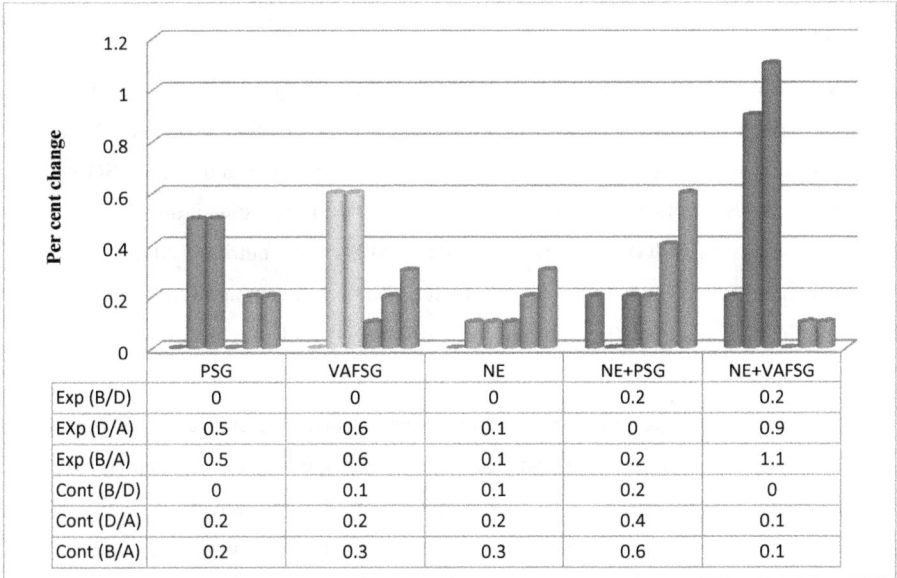

	PSG	VAFSG	NE	NE+PSG	NE+VAFSG
Exp (B/D)	0	0	0	0.2	0.2
EXp (D/A)	0.5	0.6	0.1	0	0.9
Exp (B/A)	0.5	0.6	0.1	0.2	1.1
Cont (B/D)	0	0.1	0.1	0.2	0
Cont (D/A)	0.2	0.2	0.2	0.4	0.1
Cont (B/A)	0.2	0.3	0.3	0.6	0.1

NE: The mean respective values for height in nutrition education intervention group (control and experimental) were 88.85±4.09cm, 89.95±4.08cm, 90.10±4.03cm and 90.10±4.12cm, 90.10±4.12cm 90.20±4.09cm at different stages of trial (before, during and after). Interestingly, nutrition education intervened sub-group did not show significant change at any stage of experimentation. Control sub-group presented more per cent change/improvement (0.3%) as compared to experimented sub-group (0.1%) and that too significant ($p \leq 0.05$) change at the end of the study period at B/A (0-120days) stage.

NE+PSG: Mean height values of both sub-groups (control and experimental table 4.10) represented mean change of 0.6 per cent in control sub-group as compared to NE+PSG intervened sub-group (0.2%) with statistically significant ($p \leq 0.01$) improvement after two and four months of study period. Change or improvement in control sub-group can be explained as natural or sampling fluctuations in the growth of height.

NE+VAFSG: A steady growth of 0.2, 0.9 and 1.1 per cent was noticed among NE+VAFSG supplemented sub-group during different stages of trial period. Whereas, no such change was observed in control sub-group subjects. Growth in mean height was statistically significant ($p \leq 0.01$) after two months & four months of intervention with NE+VAFSG.

Perusal of the data suggested that during the whole study period, mean changes at different stages (B/D, D/A, and B/A) were not so representative, hence may be taken as natural growth for the control sub-groups of VAFSG, NE and NE+ PSG which were however, statistically significant ($p \leq 0.01$, $p \leq 0.05$). Along with this, intervention with probiotics (PSG), value added foods (VAFSG) and nutrition education along with value added foods (NE+ VAFSG) have also shown comparatively good sign of significant change ($p \leq 0.01$) in the mid (0-60days) and end of the study period (120days).

Xu,(2019), also reported was reduction in prevalence of stunting by 27 per cent, underweight by 51 per cent and wasting by 57 per cent. A significant ($p \leq .0001$) difference was observed in the intervention group (fed with soybean-powder based complementary food) whereas no change was observed in control group.

4.5.2 Efficacy of nutrition interventions on Weight of the pre-school children

Analogue to height, weight was also measured for the control as well as experimental sub-groups. The results in kilogram have been summarized in table 4.11.

PSG: Probiotic supplemented experimental sub-group during all the three stages of intervention depicted increased in weight i.e. 4.1, 8.3 and 12.8 per cent. The paired t-test suggested highly significant ($p \leq 0.01$) improvement during all the three stages. While control sub-group of PSG reported no evidence of any significant change in weight for B/D (0-60days), D/A (60-120days), and B/A(0-120days) stages.

VAFSG: The mean weight data of value added foods supplemented sub-group at 0, 60 and 120 days represented very good improvement of 10.7, 7 and 18.5 per cent, respectively. Likewise, all the three stages have shown statistically highly significant ($p \leq 0.01$) improvement. Control sub-group mean weight values showed weight gain of 4.8 and 4.4 per cent, respectively at B/D (0-60days) and B/A (0-120days) stages with significant ($p \leq 0.01$) impact. Significant improvement among control sub-group subjects might be attributed to natural impact or change due to effect of sampling fluctuations.

Table: 4.11 Efficacy of nutrition interventions on the Weight of the pre-school children during different stages of interventions

Nutrition Interventions		Actual Increase			Mean change						t value		
		Before (0day)	During (0-60days)	After (120days)	B/D		D/A		B/A		B/D (0day)	D/A (60-120 days)	B/A (0-120 days)
					Total	%	Total	%	Total	%			
PSG	Control	9.93±0.89	9.92±0.89	10.10±0.80	0.01	0.1	0.18	1.9	0.17	1.8	1.000	1.050	1.010
	Experimental	10.35±1.30	10.78±1.24	11.67±1.26	0.43	4.1	0.89	8.3	1.32	12.8	3.48**	5.28**	6.09**
VAFSG	Control	9.45±0.60	9.90±0.91	9.87±0.73	0.45	4.8	0.03	0.3	0.42	4.4	2.93*	0.22	3.15**
	Experimental	9.70±0.86	10.74±0.89	11.50±0.90	1.04	10.7	0.76	7	1.8	18.5	6.79**	5.39**	11.19**
NE	Control	10.05±1.09	10.30±1.30	10.31±1.07	0.25	2.5	0.01	0.1	0.26	2.6	2.51*	0.06	1.628
	Experimental	9.93±1.05	10.16±0.92	10.82±1.03	0.23	2.4	0.66	6.5	0.9	9	2.36*	4.21**	5.70**
NE+PSG	Control	9.80±1.00	9.80±0.69	9.70±0.65	0	0	0.1	1	0.1	1	0	1	0.62
	Experimental	10.61±1.48	12.05±1.44	12.05±1.44	1.45	13.6	0	0	1.45	13.6	12.6**	0	12.61**
NE+ VAFSG	Control	9.68±0.81	9.58±0.81	9.78±0.75	0.1	1	0.2	2.1	0.1	1	1.7	1.45	0.67
	Experimental	10.09±0.77	11.14±0.92	11.92±0.86	1.05	10.4	0.78	7	1.83	18.1	7.76**	6.60**	14.98**

**significant at $p \leq 0.01$, *significant at $p \leq 0.05$

Control– No Intervention

PSG- Probiotic supplemented group; **VAFSG** –Value-added food supplemented group; **NE** –Nutrition education; **NE+PSG-** Nutrition education+ Probiotic supplemented group; **NE +VAFSG** – Nutrition education + value -added food supplemented group

B/D – Before / During **D/A**- During/ After **B/A**– Before/ After

Fig.4.32 Mean Weight of pre-school children during different stages of nutrition interventions

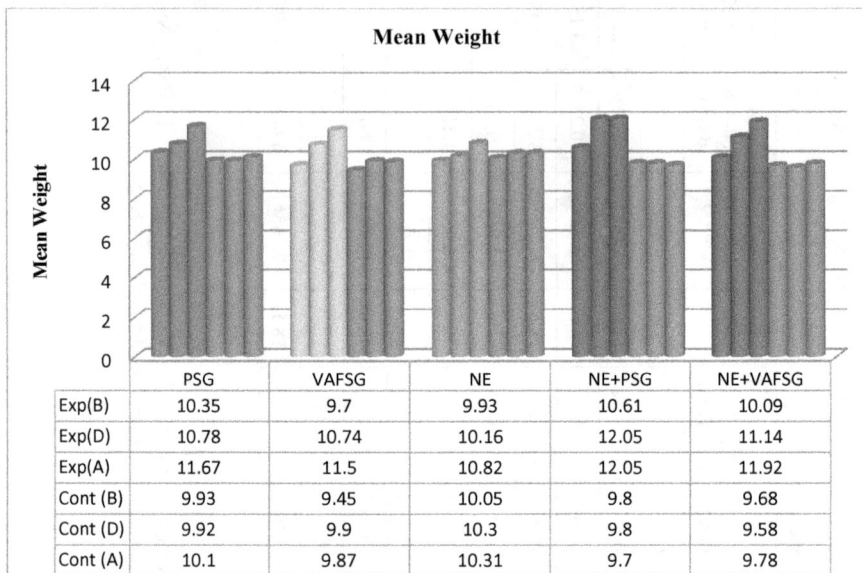

Mean Weight

	PSG	VAFSG	NE	NE+PSG	NE+VAFSG
Exp(B)	10.35	9.7	9.93	10.61	10.09
Exp(D)	10.78	10.74	10.16	12.05	11.14
Exp(A)	11.67	11.5	10.82	12.05	11.92
Cont (B)	9.93	9.45	10.05	9.8	9.68
Cont (D)	9.92	9.9	10.3	9.8	9.58
Cont (A)	10.1	9.87	10.31	9.7	9.78

Fig.4.33 Per cent change in Weight of the pre-school children before during and after intervention

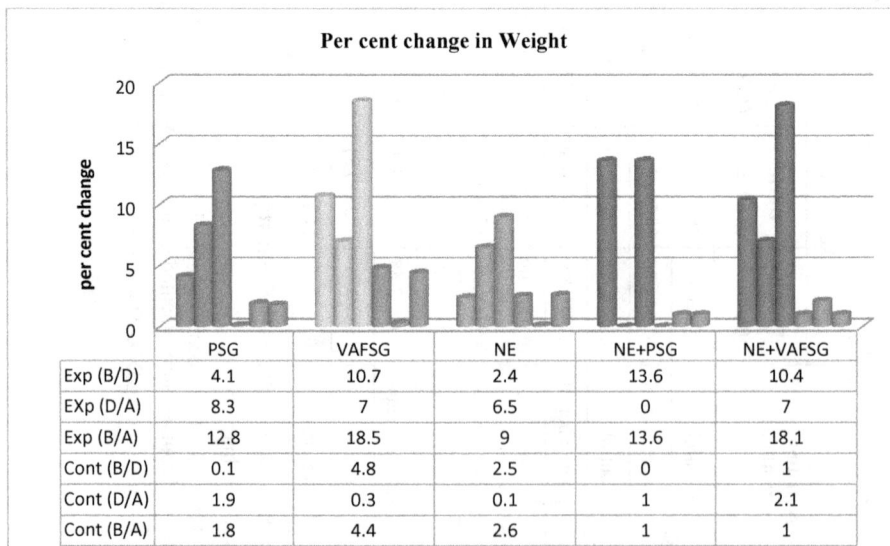

Per cent change in Weight

	PSG	VAFSG	NE	NE+PSG	NE+VAFSG
Exp (B/D)	4.1	10.7	2.4	13.6	10.4
EXp (D/A)	8.3	7	6.5	0	7
Exp (B/A)	12.8	18.5	9	13.6	18.1
Cont (B/D)	0.1	4.8	2.5	0	1
Cont (D/A)	1.9	0.3	0.1	1	2.1
Cont (B/A)	1.8	4.4	2.6	1	1

NE: The observed mean values for experiment and control sub-groups of nutrition education group were 9.93±1.05kg, 10.16±0.92kg, 10.82±1.03kg, and 10.05±1.09kg, 10.30±1.30kg, 10.31±1.07kg at before, during and after trial period, respectively. The mean per cent change in weight for experimental sub-group was 9 per cent as compared to only 2.6 per cent for control sub-group. Experiment sub-group subjects showed significant (p≤0.01) weight gain at all the stages of nutrition education intervention period depicting quite good impact of nutrition education. However control sub-group showed significant (p≤0.05) effects at the initial (0day) stage only which can be explained on natural growth basis.

NE+PSG: The nutrition education and probiotic supplemented experiment and control sub-group's mean weight for all the three phases of experiment were 10.61±1.48kg, 12.05±1.44kg, 12.05±1.44kg and 9.80±1.00kg, 9.80±0.69kg, 9.70±0.65kg, respectively. Mean per cent change in weight for the experiment sub-group after 120 days was 13.6 per cent as compared to only 1 per cent for control sub-group. A significant (p≤0.01) improvement was noticed on NE+PSG supplementation after 60 days and 120 days as compared to non significant change among control subgroup subjects.

NE+VAFSG: The data calculated for NE+VAFG experiment sub-group demonstrated the mean per cent change in weight gain of 10.4, 7.0 and 18.1, respectively at initial, mid and completion of intervention trial. Highly significant gain (p≤0.01) was noticed at the intervention stages. Whereas, the observed mean weight for the control sub-group i.e. 9.68±0.81kg, 9.58±0.81kg and 9.78±0.75kg before, during and after, respectively represented negligible change at all stages.

Further data analysis suggested almost same pattern of per cent weight gain for VAFSG (18.5%) and NE+VAFSG (18.1%) supplemented group followed by NE+PSG (13.6%) and PSG (12.8%). Correspondingly, significant improvement in weight was noticed among the experimental sub-groups of PSG, VAFSG, NE, NE+VAFSG at all stages of trial. However, control sub-group of VAFSG and NE also showed significant impact at B/D & B/A and B/D respectively. This can be explained as natural growth gain process.

Study reported by Wang *et.al* (2017) is in line with present findings. They observed that soybean value-added food played a vital role for reducing the prevalence of stunting and underweight among children aged 12-23 months. The study further concluded that value-added food with imparting nutrition education improved the dietary intake and reduced the prevalence of malnutrition. Khader and Maheshwari, (2012) also revealed that amylase-rich malted mixes supplementation for period of 120 days increased the weight of pre-school children significantly. The findings of Mahfuz *et.al,* (2014) also reported that feeding with ready to use food to experimental group showed a significant weight gain whereas control group did not show any change in weight of the children. A review study by Onubi, (2015) concluded that probiotics were helpful in gain weight and height of malnourished children. It further added that local available food must be supplemented with probiotics to improve the anthropometric parameters.

4.5.3 Efficacy of nutrition interventions on BMI of the pre-school children

BMI was measured as per indicators given in tables 4.10 and 4.11 on height and weight of the sample subgroups under different allotted nutrition interventions, and the results are summarized in table 4.12.

PSG: Mean BMI values for experimental and control sub-groups of PSG as evident in table 4.12 indicated continuous improvement of 3.7, 7.9, 11.9 percent and 0.8, 1.0, 1.8 per cent in body mass index respectively at 0, 60 and 120 days. Likewise, statistically significant ($p \leq 0.01$) increment was observed among probiotic supplemented sub-group at all the three stages of analysis (0, 60 &120 days), whereas no significant change was observed in control sub-group to whom no probiotic was fed.

VAFSG: The mean values calculated in respect of BMI kg/m^2 for experimental sub-group were $12.91\pm0.95kg/m^2$, $14.21\pm1.06kg/m^2$, and 15.13 ± 1.04 kg/m^2 and for control sub-group were $12.63\pm1.18kg/m^2$, $12.63\pm1.18kg/m^2$ and $12.53\pm0.81kg/m^2$, before, during and after the feeding trial, respectively. Both the sub-groups represented same pattern of increment during different stages of trial, however per cent increment was

Table: 4.12 Efficacy of nutrition interventions on the BMI of the pre-school children during different stages of interventions

Nutrition Interventions		Actual Increase			Mean change							t value		
		Before (0day)	During (60days)	After (120days)	B/D		D/A		B/A			B/D (0-60days)	D/A (60-120days)	B/A (0-120days)
					Total	%	Total	%	Total	%				
PSG	Control	11.84±0.92	11.93±0.88	12.06±1.05	0.09	0.8	0.12	1	0.21	1.8		1.000	0.504	0.970
	Experimental	12.96±1.11	13.44±1.08	14.50±1.12	0.48	3.7	1.06	7.9	1.54	11.9		2.97**	3.97**	4.49**
VAFSG	Control	12.63±1.18	12.63±1.18	12.53±0.81	0.56	4.6	0.1	0.8	0.45	3.7		2.89**	0.6	2.68**
	Experimental	12.91±0.95	14.21±1.06	15.13±1.04	1.31	10.1	0.92	6.5	2.22	17.2		6.27**	3.82**	10.76**
N.E	Control	12.42±0.67	12.69±0.88	12.68±0.76	0.27	2.1	0.01	0.1	0.26	2.1		2.31*	0.04	1.35
	Experimental	12.21±0.88	12.47±0.79	13.15±0.55	0.25	2.1	0.69	5.5	0.94	7.7		1.99	3.92**	5.20**
NE+ PSG	Control	12.30±1.00	12.29±0.95	12.07±1.13	0.01	0.1	0.21	1.7	0.22	1.8		0.06	1.55	1.05
	Experimental	12.56±0.85	14.22±0.91	14.22±0.91	1.66	13.22	0	0	1.66	13.2		9.29**	0	9.29**
NE+ VAFSG	Control	12.18±1.04	12.06±1.07	12.30±1.00	0.12	1	0.24	2	0.11	0.9		1.65	1.32	0.59
	Experimental	12.89±0.75	14.16±0.90	15.04±0.69	1.27	9.9	0.87	6.2	2.15	16.7		8.56**	5.92**	13.39**

**significant at p≤0.01, *significant at p≤ 0.05

CONTROL– No Intervention

PSG- Probiotic supplemented group; **VAFSG** –Value-added food supplemented group; **NE** –Nutrition education; **NE+PSG**- Nutrition education+ Probiotic supplemented group; **NE +VAFSG** – Nutrition education + value -added food supplemented group

B/D – Before / During **D/A**- During / After **B/A**– Before/ After

much more in experimental sub-group (17.2%) as compared to control sub-group (3.7%) on the completion of trial period (120days). Correspondingly, statistically significant (p≤0.01) change in BMI parameters was observed for both sub-groups at all the three stages except D/A stage of control sub-group. Control sub-group did not report much improvement i.e. only 4.6 and 3.7 even though; t static values showed significant (p≤0.01) change which might be because of standard error or sampling fluctuations.

NE: A steady increment in mean per cent BMI values (2.1%, 5.5% and 7.7%) of nutrition education intervened sub-group was noticed (Table 4.12). Control sub-group (to whom no nutrition education was given) represented 2.1 per cent increment at initial and final stage of trial period, but t static showed significant effect only in B/D which can be explained as normal growth or sample fluctuation error. Further, among experiment sub-group subjects, an improvement of 5.5 and 7.7 per cent analyzed as significant (p≤0.01) statistically, symbolized efficacy of nutrition education intervention after 60 and 120 days of trial period.

NE+PSG: NE+PSG group was intervened experimental sub-group's respective mean BMI values before, during and after trial period i.e.12.56±0.85kg/m^2, 14.22±0.91kg/m^2 and 14.22±0.91kg/m^2 symbolized mean improvement of 13.2 per cent at the starting and end of intervention. Correspondingly, improvement in BMI was calculated as statistically significant (p≤0.01) at both the stages. Control sub-group subjects mean BMI values also indicated improvement but that was very less (1.8%), hence non significant statistically. Analysis of the data further, strengthened the impact of NE+PSG on mean BMI status.

NE+VAFSG: Mean per cent change of 9.9, 6.2 and 16.7 in BMI for experiment sub-group subjects exhibited statistical significant change (p≤0.01) at all the stages of analysis as represented in table (4.12). Whereas, negligible (1.0, 2.0, 0.9) per cent change in BMI values of control sub-group subjects advocates efficacy of combined therapy of nutrition education along with feeding of value added foods on improving BMI status. Further analysis of the data represented that maximum impact was observed with VAFSG (17.2%) followed by NE+VAFSG (16.7%), NE+PSG (13.2%), PSG (11.9%) and NE (7.7%). Hence, VAFSG was inferred as

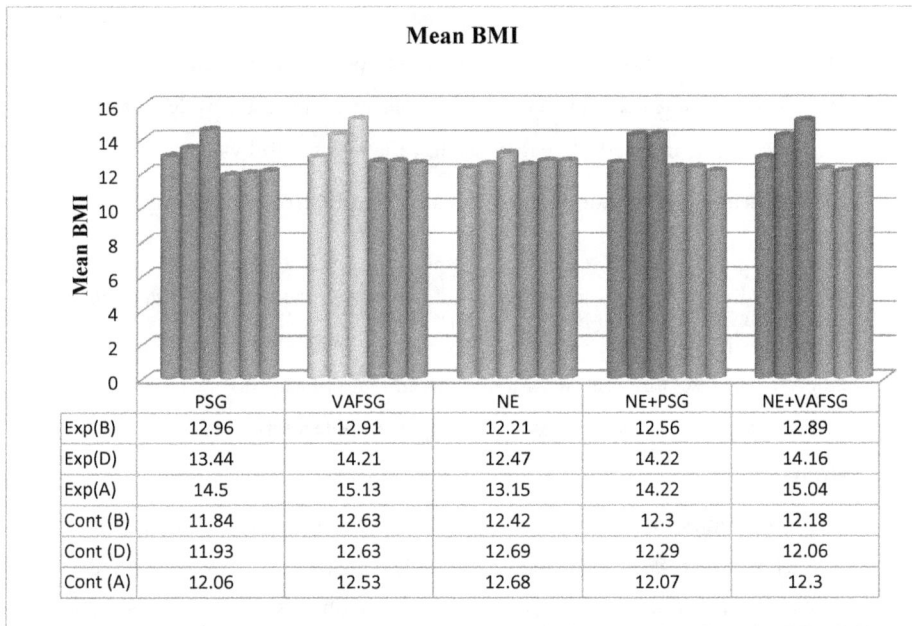

Mean BMI

	PSG	VAFSG	NE	NE+PSG	NE+VAFSG
Exp(B)	12.96	12.91	12.21	12.56	12.89
Exp(D)	13.44	14.21	12.47	14.22	14.16
Exp(A)	14.5	15.13	13.15	14.22	15.04
Cont (B)	11.84	12.63	12.42	12.3	12.18
Cont (D)	11.93	12.63	12.69	12.29	12.06
Cont (A)	12.06	12.53	12.68	12.07	12.3

Fig.4.34 Mean BMI of pre-school children during different stages of nutrition
interventions

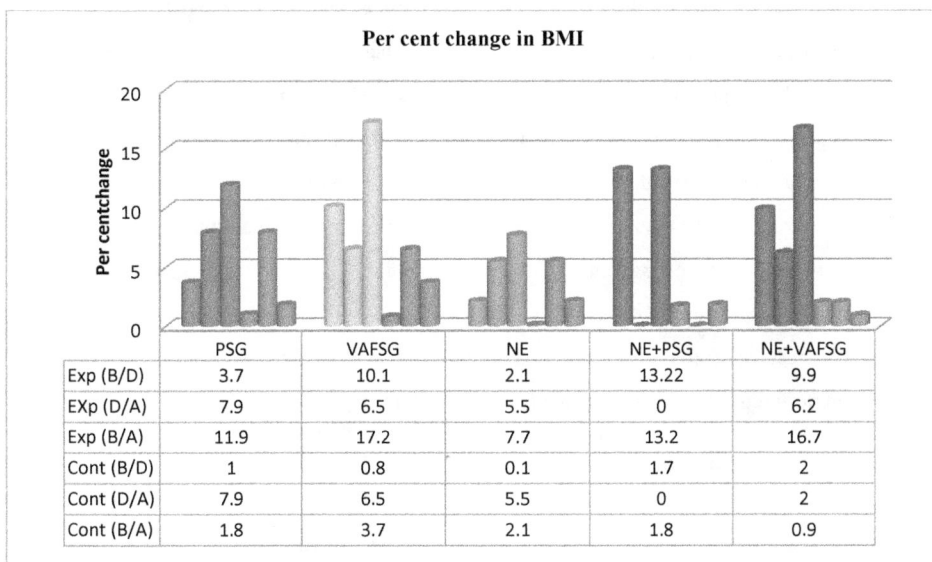

Per cent change in BMI

	PSG	VAFSG	NE	NE+PSG	NE+VAFSG
Exp (B/D)	3.7	10.1	2.1	13.22	9.9
EXp (D/A)	7.9	6.5	5.5	0	6.2
Exp (B/A)	11.9	17.2	7.7	13.2	16.7
Cont (B/D)	1	0.8	0.1	1.7	2
Cont (D/A)	7.9	6.5	5.5	0	2
Cont (B/A)	1.8	3.7	2.1	1.8	0.9

Fig. 4.35 Per cent change in BMI of the pre-school children before during and
after intervention

97

most effective intervention treatment. Perusal of the facts further revealed that the outcome pattern of the experimentation trial in respect of BMI is similar to that of analysis of weight under study. Hence in present study, impact of weight variation was noticed to be more effective than height variations on BMI values.

4.5.4 Efficacy of nutrition interventions on Head Circumference of the pre-school children

The head circumference is a vital parameter to monitor the growth of brain during the growth period of the children. The head circumference of all the selected children for five different nutrition intervention groups was recorded before (0day), during (0-60day) and after (120days) the intervention period with their subgroups and the result are depicted in the table 4.13.

The mean values of head circumference for PSG experimental sub-group were 46.45±1.50cm, 46.45±1.50cm and 46.67±1.27cm at 0 days, 60 days and 120 days of feeding intervention, respectively. With overall 0.5 per cent increment, significant ($p \leq 0.05$) change was observed after 2 months and 4 months of the PSG trial. All the sub-groups of different interventions represented almost negligible mean percent change in head circumference , hence non-significant change was noticed except for PSG experiment sub-group which might have been due to measurement error or otherwise. The study concluded that there was no effect of any nutrition intervention on the development or growth of head circumference in the sample unit. López-Alonso *et.al*, (2021) carried out a Quantitative study and intervened the respondents with complementary feeding supplemented with amaranth flour to the experimental group whereas control group with no feeding. The results of the study revealed after three months of experiment that head circumference had no significant ($p \geq 0.05$) difference.

Table: 4.13 Efficacy of nutrition interventions on the Head Circumference of the pre-school children during different stages of interventions

Experimental Groups		Actual Increase			Mean change							t value		
		Before	During	After	B/D		D/A		B/A			B/D	D/A	B/A
					Total	%	Total	%	Total	%				
PSG	Control	45.70±1.72	45.70±1.72	45.80±1.76	0	0	0.1	0.2	0.1	0.2		0.000	1.450	1.450
	Experimental	46.45±1.50	46.45±1.50	46.67±1.27	0	0	0.21	0.5	0.21	0.5		0	2.16*	2.16*
VAFSG	Control	46.95±0.88	47±0.85	47.05±0.88	0.05	0.1	0.05	0.1	0.1	0.2		1	1	1.45
	Experimental	47.40±0.50	47.35±0.48	47.50±0.51	0.05	0.1	0.15	0.3	0.1	0.2		1	1.83	1
N.E	Control	47.45±1.60	47.45±.1.60	47.45±1.60	0	0	0	0	0	0		0	0	0
	Experimental	45.63±1.58	45.63±1.58	45.68±1.61	0	0	0.05	0.01	0.05	0		0	1	1
NE+PSG	Control	46.55±1.46	46.60±1.50	46.70±1.41	0.05	0.1	0.1	0.2	0.15	0.3		1	1.45	1.83
	Experimental	45.25±2.42	45.25±2.42	45.25±2.42	0	0	0	0	0	0		0	0	0
NE+VAFSG	Control	46.40±1.50	46.40±1.50	46.40±1.50	0	0	0	0	0	0		0	0	0
	Experimental	47±0.97	46.95±0.94	46.95±0.94	0.05	0.1	0	0	0.05	0.1		1	0	1

*significant at p≤ 0.05

CONTROL– No Intervention

PSG- Probiotic supplemented group; VAFSG –Value-added food supplemented group NE –Nutrition education; NE+PSG- Nutrition education+ Probiotic supplemented group; NE +VAFSG – Nutrition education + value -added food supplemented group

B/D – Before / During D/A– During/ After B/A– Before/ After

Fig.4.36 Mean Head Circumference of pre-school children during different stages of nutrition interventions

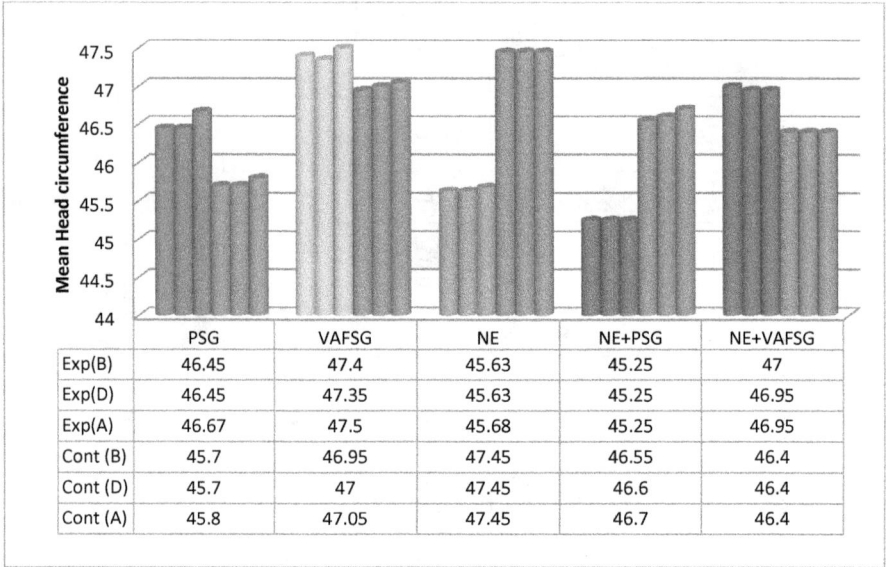

	PSG	VAFSG	NE	NE+PSG	NE+VAFSG
Exp(B)	46.45	47.4	45.63	45.25	47
Exp(D)	46.45	47.35	45.63	45.25	46.95
Exp(A)	46.67	47.5	45.68	45.25	46.95
Cont (B)	45.7	46.95	47.45	46.55	46.4
Cont (D)	45.7	47	47.45	46.6	46.4
Cont (A)	45.8	47.05	47.45	46.7	46.4

Fig. 4.37 Per cent change in Head circumference of the pre-school children before during and after intervention

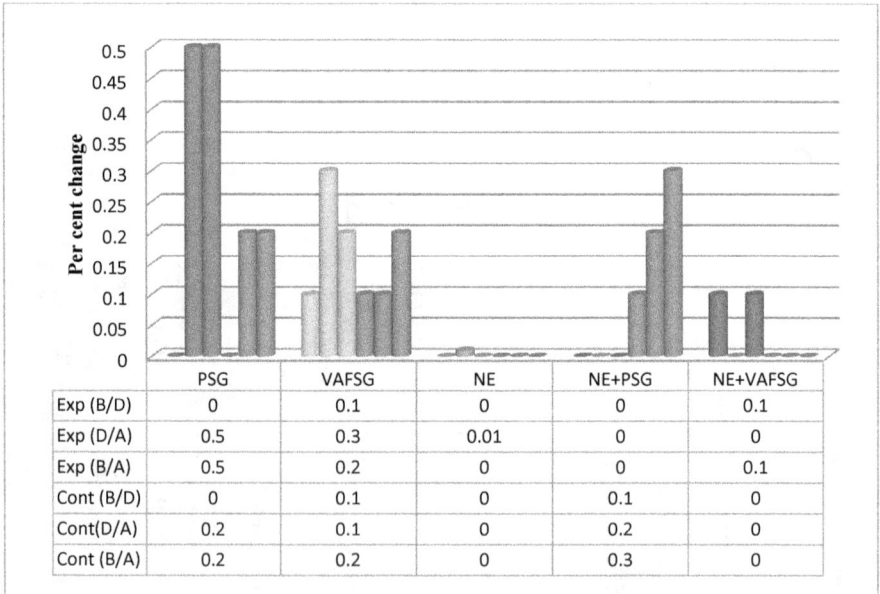

	PSG	VAFSG	NE	NE+PSG	NE+VAFSG
Exp (B/D)	0	0.1	0	0	0.1
Exp (D/A)	0.5	0.3	0.01	0	0
Exp (B/A)	0.5	0.2	0	0	0.1
Cont (B/D)	0	0.1	0	0.1	0
Cont(D/A)	0.2	0.1	0	0.2	0
Cont (B/A)	0.2	0.2	0	0.3	0

4.5.5 Efficacy of nutrition interventions on Chest Circumference of the pre-school children

Chest circumference was considered as one of the parameters to study anthropometric evaluation based on the five nutrition interventions, namely PSG, VAFSG, NE, NE+PSG, and NE+VAFSG for two sub-groups (control and experiment). The data generated through the experimentation has been summarized in table 4.14.

PSG: The observed mean values of chest circumference experimental sub-group at before (0day), during (60days) and after (120days) study period were 47.60±1.69cm, 47.65±1.63cm and 47.80±1.67cm respectively depicting mean per cent change of 0.4, corresponding to significant ($p \leq 0.05$) change but only after 120 days of trial. The control sub-group did not show any significant growth in chest circumference during the entire trial period.

VAFSG, NE, and NE+PSG: As is clear from the analysis (Table 4.14) that during the experimentation period (0-120 days), VAFSG, NE, and NE+PSG have not shown any improvement in the chest circumference of pre-school children under study. The mean values for all the subgroups were of almost same order. The static analysis is evident that there was no significant increment in any of the subgroup.

NE+VAFSG: Interestingly, control sub-group has shown significant changes for D/A ($p \leq 0.05$) and B/A ($p \leq 0.01$) with 0.7 per cent increment and in contrast, the experiment sub-group did not show any changes at al. However, significant change in the control sub-group may be due to some natural growth or effect of sampling distribution.

Almost a similar trend of mean percentage change was observed among the control and experimental sub-groups of all the intervention groups except for control sub-group of NE+VAFSG and experiment sub-group of PSG. Significant ($p \leq 0.01$) change in these two sub-groups can be explained as on basis of process of natural growth or sampling distribution.

Table: 4.14 Efficacy of nutrition interventions on the Chest Circumference of the pre-school children during different stages of interventions

Experimental Groups		Actual Increase			Mean change						t value		
		Before	During	After	B/D		D/A		B/A		B/D	D/A	B/A
					Total	%	Total	%	Total	%			
PSG	Control	46.90±1.44	46.90±1.44	46.95±1.50	0	0	0.05	0.1	0.05	0.1	0.000	1.000	1.000
	Experimental	47.60±1.69	47.65±1.63	47.80±1.67	0.05	0.1	0.15	0.3	0.2	0.4	1	1.83	2.17*
VAFSG	Control	47.40±0.94	47.40±0.94	47.50±0.88	0	0	0.1	0.2	0.1	0.2	0	1.45	1.45
	Experimental	48.75±0.63	48.85±0.74	48.90±0.78	0.1	0.2	0.05	0.1	0.15	0.3	1.45	1	1.3
N.E	Control	46.65±1.87	46.65±1.87	46.80±2.01	0	0	0.15	0.3	0.15	0.3	0	1.83	1.83
	Experimental	46.55±1.39	46.60±1.42	46.70±1.55	0.05	0.1	0.1	0.2	0.15	0.3	1	1.45	1.83
NE+PSG	Control	46.35±0.98	46.35±0.98	46.45±0.99	0	0	0.1	0.2	0.1	0.2	0	1.45	1.45
	Experimental	46.65±2.231	46.65±2.231	46.65±2.231	0	0	0	0	0	0	0	0	0
NE+VAFSG	Control	47.70±1.17	47.75±1.25	48.05±1.35	0.05	0.1	0.3	0.6	0.35	0.7	1	2.85**	3.199**
	Experimental	47.35±1.84	47.35±1.84	47.35±1.84	0	0	0	0	0	0	0	0	0

**Significant at p≤0.01 * Significant at p≤0.05

CONTROL– No Intervention

PSG- Probiotic supplemented group; VAFSG –Value-added food supplemented group;

NE –Nutrition education; NE+PSG- Nutrition education+ Probiotic supplemented group; NE +VAFSG – Nutrition education + value - added food supplemented group B/D – Before / During D/A- During/ After B/A– Before/ After

Fig. 4.38 Mean Chest Circumference of pre-school children during different stages of nutrition interventions

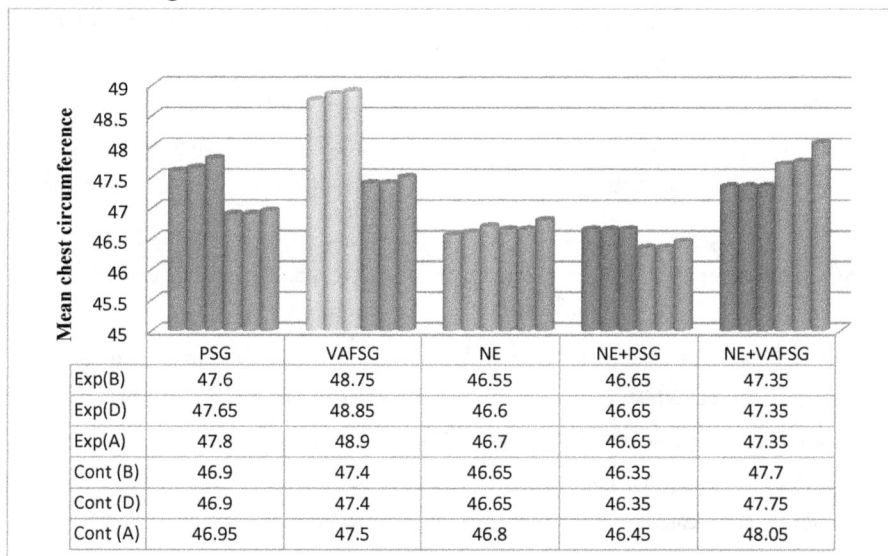

	PSG	VAFSG	NE	NE+PSG	NE+VAFSG
Exp(B)	47.6	48.75	46.55	46.65	47.35
Exp(D)	47.65	48.85	46.6	46.65	47.35
Exp(A)	47.8	48.9	46.7	46.65	47.35
Cont (B)	46.9	47.4	46.65	46.35	47.7
Cont (D)	46.9	47.4	46.65	46.35	47.75
Cont (A)	46.95	47.5	46.8	46.45	48.05

Fig. 4.39 Per cent change in Chest Circumference of the pre-school children before during and after intervention

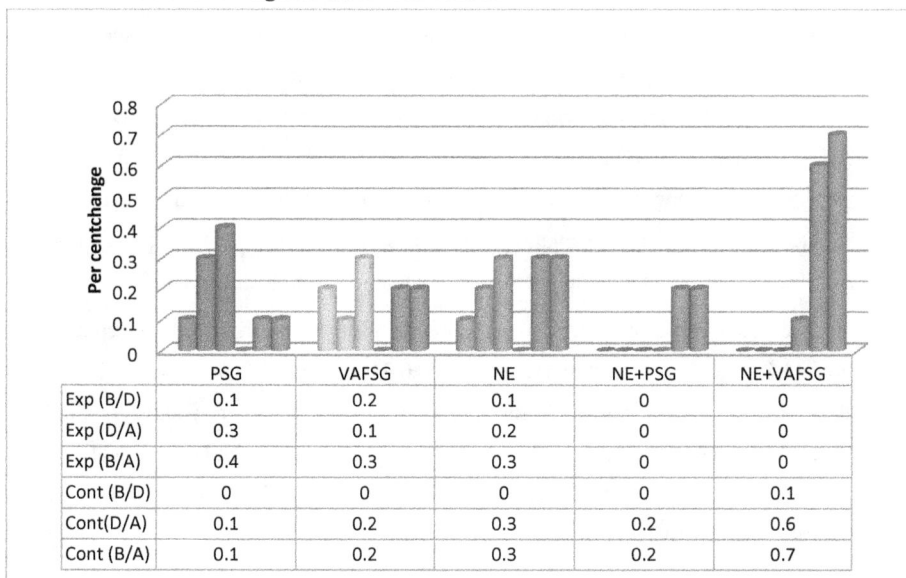

	PSG	VAFSG	NE	NE+PSG	NE+VAFSG
Exp (B/D)	0.1	0.2	0.1	0	0
Exp (D/A)	0.3	0.1	0.2	0	0
Exp (B/A)	0.4	0.3	0.3	0	0
Cont (B/D)	0	0	0	0	0.1
Cont(D/A)	0.1	0.2	0.3	0.2	0.6
Cont (B/A)	0.1	0.2	0.3	0.2	0.7

4.5.6 Efficacy of nutrition interventions on Arm Circumference of the pre-school children

Arm circumference has been considered a quite vital indicator to study the efficacy of nutrition interventions due to many biological reasons. The mean values, mean percent change and t static were examined for both the control and experimental sub-groups before, during and after the trial period. The experiment was continued for 120 days, and the data generated has been statistically analyzed and presented in table 4.15.

PSG: It was interesting to note that arm circumference in the case of the control sub-group has shown growth during (60days) as well as after the intervention period (0-120days). The mean changes for B/D, D/A, and B/A presented constant growth as 2.3, 6.6 and 9 percent. While comparing the changes through the application of paired t-test, all three stages, namely B/D, D/A, and B/A, were significant at 1 per cent since the control sub-group has not been given any extra nutrition, the changes may be due to other external causes. Experiment sub-group depicted mean changes of 11.7 per cent, which was also significant (p≤0.01) through paired t-test at 1 per cent level of significance. It indicates that PSG has shown the actual effect in the experiment sub-group.

VAFSG: The observed respective mean values of arm circumference as shown in table 4.15 indicated same trend of improvement (4% and 4.3%) among both sub-groups during entire studied period. Further analysis suggested the change at D/A (60-120days) and B/A (0-120days) t values were statistically significant (p≤0.05 and p≤0.01). As the change was almost of equal order in both the sub-groups, real effect of value added foods supplementation cannot be safely attributed. Hence, change may be credited to natural or external factors associated with sample under study.

NE: The mean values of nutrition education subgroups (experimental and control) were 11.88±0.64cm, 11.78±0.61cm, 12.15±0.74cm and 10.45±0.94cm, 10.60± 1.04cm, 10.70±1.08cm before, during and after the trial period, respectively. Mean per cent improvement of 2.4 and 2.3 was noticed among control and experiment sub-groups, respectively with statistically, significant (p≤0.05 and p≤0.01) improvement was observed for B/A (control) and D/A (experimental).

Table: 4.15 Efficacy of nutrition interventions on the Arm Circumference of the pre-school children during different stages of interventions

Experimental Groups		Actual Increase			Mean change						t value		
		Before (0day)	During (60days)	After (120days)	B/D		D/A		B/A		B/D (0-60 days)	D/A (60-120 days)	B/A (0-120 days)
					Total	%	Total	%	Total	%			
PSG	Control	11.93±0.89	12.20±0.67	13±0.99	0.28	2.3	0.8	6.6	1.08	9	2.84**	3.38**	4.24**
	Experimental	11.55±0.88	11.55±0.88	12.90±0.96	0	0	1.35	11.7	1.35	11.7	0	4.92**	4.92**
VAFSG	Control	9.90±0.64	10.05±0.51	10.30±0.65	0.15	1.5	0.25	2.5	0.4	4	1.37	2.51**	2.99**
	Experimental	11.73±0.71	11.83±0.67	12.23±0.57	0.1	0.9	0.4	3.4	0.5	4.3	1.45	3.55**	4.35**
N.E	Control	10.45±0.94	10.60±1.04	10.70±1.08	0.15	1.4	0.1	0.9	0.25	2.4	1.83	1.45	2.51**
	Experimental	11.88±0.64	11.78±0.61	12.15±0.74	0.1	0.8	0.38	3.2	0.28	2.3	1	2.88**	1.92
NE+PSG	Control	11.10±0.71	11.25±0.71	11.50±0.76	0.15	1.4	0.25	2.2	0.4	3.6	1.83	2.51**	3.55**
	Experimental	12.10±0.71	12.70±0.80	12.80±0.89	0.6	5	0.1	0.8	0.7	5.8	3.94**	1.45	4.76**
NE+ VAFSG	Control	10.89±0.87	10.94±0.96	10.89±0.87	0.05	0.4	0.05	0.5	0.01	0	0.4	0.56	0.03
	Experimental	12.08±0.65	12.20±0.59	12.43±0.63	0.13	1	0.23	1.8	0.35	2.9	1.22	1.75	3.19**

**significant at p≤0.01, *significant at p≤ 0.05

CONTROL– No Intervention

PSG- Probiotic supplemented group; VAFSG –Value-added food supplemented group; NE –Nutrition education; NE+PSG- Nutrition education+ Probiotic supplemented group; NE +VAFSG – Nutrition education + value -added food supplemented group

B/D – Before / During D/A- During/ After B/A– Before/ After

Fig. 4.40 Mean Arm Circumference of pre-school children during different stages of nutrition interventions

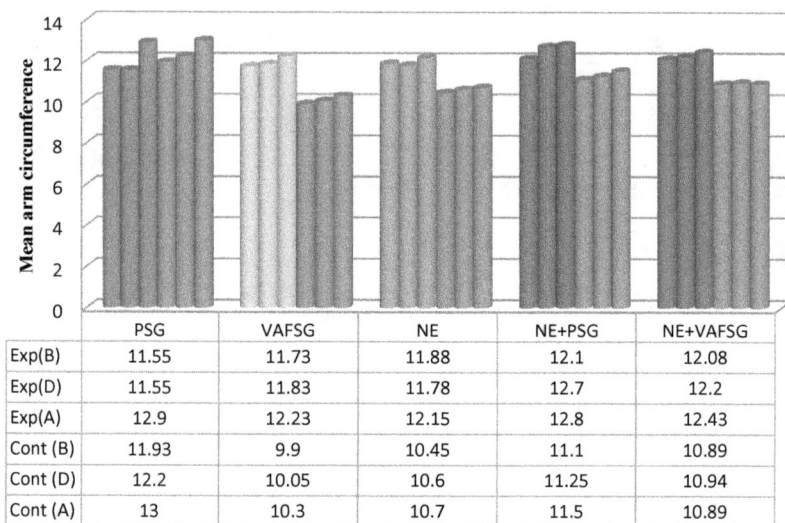

	PSG	VAFSG	NE	NE+PSG	NE+VAFSG
Exp(B)	11.55	11.73	11.88	12.1	12.08
Exp(D)	11.55	11.83	11.78	12.7	12.2
Exp(A)	12.9	12.23	12.15	12.8	12.43
Cont (B)	11.93	9.9	10.45	11.1	10.89
Cont (D)	12.2	10.05	10.6	11.25	10.94
Cont (A)	13	10.3	10.7	11.5	10.89

Fig. 4.41 Per cent change in Arm Circumference of the pre-school children before during and after intervention

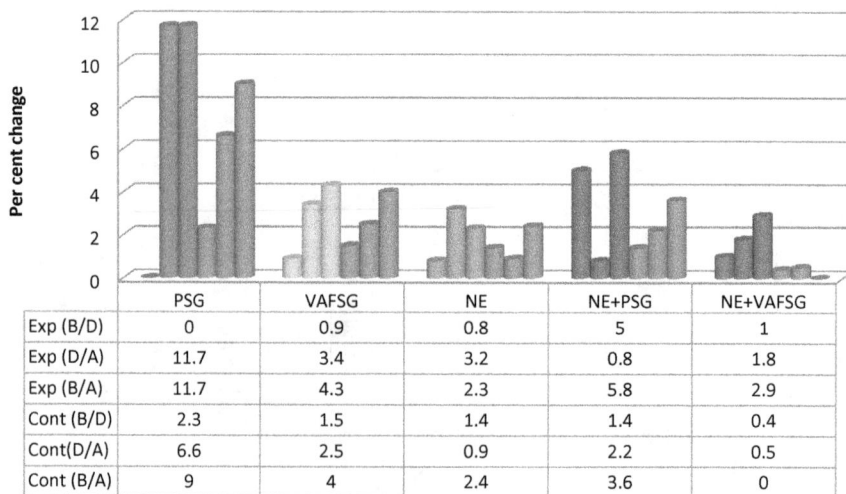

	PSG	VAFSG	NE	NE+PSG	NE+VAFSG
Exp (B/D)	0	0.9	0.8	5	1
Exp (D/A)	11.7	3.4	3.2	0.8	1.8
Exp (B/A)	11.7	4.3	2.3	5.8	2.9
Cont (B/D)	2.3	1.5	1.4	1.4	0.4
Cont(D/A)	6.6	2.5	0.9	2.2	0.5
Cont (B/A)	9	4	2.4	3.6	0

NE+PSG: The nutrition education and probiotic supplemented sub-groups revealed mean arm circumference values in increasing order (table 4.15) at before, during and after intervention trial period. Experiment sub-group showed mean per cent change of 5.8 as compared to 3.6 per cent for control sub-group and statistically, both sub-groups represented significant improvement ($p \leq 0.05$ and $p \leq 0.01$) respectively.

NE+VAFSG: The mean arm circumference data of experimental sub-group collected before, during and after the experiment were 12.08±0.65cm, 12.20±0.59cm and 12.43±0.63cm, respectively. Experiment sub-group showed significant change ($p \leq 0.01$) with 2.9 per cent gain as compared to zero improvement among control sub-group subjects at the end of the intervention trail period.

Maximum gain in arm circumference was noticed among the experiment sub-groups of PSG (11.7%) followed by NE+PSG (5.8%) and VAFSG (4.3%). Significant change ($P \leq 0.01$) among the control sub-groups of PSG, VAFSF and NE+PSG indicated comparatively no such good impact of nutrition interventions on improving arm circumference among the experiment sub-groups.

4.5.7 Efficacy of nutrition interventions on Subcapsular Skinfold Thickness of the pre-school children

Measurements were also recorded for subcapsular skinfold thickness in respect of control as well as experiment sub-groups. Nutrition interventions like PSG, VAFSG, NE, NE+PSG, and NE+VAFSG were introduced in respect of the experimental sub-group only. The effects of nutrition interventions on subscapular skin fold thickness before, during, and after study period were recorded and presented in table 4.16. Most of the interventions under study have not shown any efficacy of nutrition interventions on subscapular skin fold thickness except VAFSG and NE +VAFSG. VAFSG and NE+VAFSG experiment sub-group children indicated mean change of 7.8 and 3.4 per cent, respectively as compared to only 0.2 and zero per cent by respective control sub-group at the end of studied period. Statistically, significant improvement was noted in VAFGS (D/A & B/A) and NE+VAFSG (B/D, D/A &B/A) experiment sub-group. Thus efficacy of supplementation with value added foods may affect the subcapsular skin fold thickness in the long run. Consequently, VAFSG either independent or along with nutrition education can be considered effective for its efficacy on subcapsular skin fold thickness improvement among the experiment subjects.

Table: 4.16 Efficacy of nutrition interventions on the Subscapular Skinfold Thickness of the pre-school children during different stages of interventions

Experimental Groups		Actual Increase			Mean change						t value		
		Before (0day)	During (60days)	After (120days)	B/D		D/A		B/A		B/D (0-60 days)	D/A (60-120 days)	B/A (0-120 days)
					Total	%	Total	%	Total	%			
PSG	Control	4.40±0.788	4.38±0.81	4.36±0.81	0.02	0.5	0.02	0.3	0.04	0.8	0.890	0.150	0.380
	Experimental	3.89±0.49	3.92±0.48	4.02±0.48	0.03	0.8	0.1	2.6	0.13	3.3	1.37	1.63	2.02
VAFSG	Control	2.89±0.38	2.89±0.38	2.90±0.38	0	0	0	0.2	0	0.2	0	1	1
	Experimental	2.88±0.71	2.86±0.61	3.10±0.61	0.02	0.7	0.25	8.6	0.23	7.8	0.25	2.92**	2.12*
N.E	Control	3.26±0.39	3.26±0.38	3.27±0.40	0.01	0.2	0.01	0.3	0.02	0.5	1	1.45	1.83
	Experimental	3.59±0.74	3.38±0.86	3.46±0.76	0.21	5.9	0.08	2.5	0.13	3.5	1.8	1.39	1.12
NE+PSG	Control	3.79±0.35	3.82±0.36	3.84±0.34	0.03	0.8	0.02	0.5	0.05	1.3	1.37	1.17	2.12**
	Experimental	2.86±0.45	2.93±0.41	2.93±0.41	0.07	2.3	0	0	0.07	2.3	0.97	0	0.97
NE+VAFSG	Control	3.57±0.34	3.57±0.34	3.57±0.34	0	0	0	0	0	0	0	0	0
	Experimental	3.08±0.63	3.11±0.60	3.18±0.60	0.04	1.1	0.07	2.3	0.11	3.4	2.10*	2.20*	3.12**

**significant at $p \leq 0.01$, *significant at $p \leq 0.05$

CONTROL– No Intervention

PSG- Probiotic supplemented group; VAFSG –Value-added food supplemented group; NE –Nutrition education; NE+PSG- Nutrition education+ Probiotic supplemented group; NE +VAFSG – Nutrition education + value -added food supplemented group

B/D – Before / During D/A- During/ After B/A– Before/ After

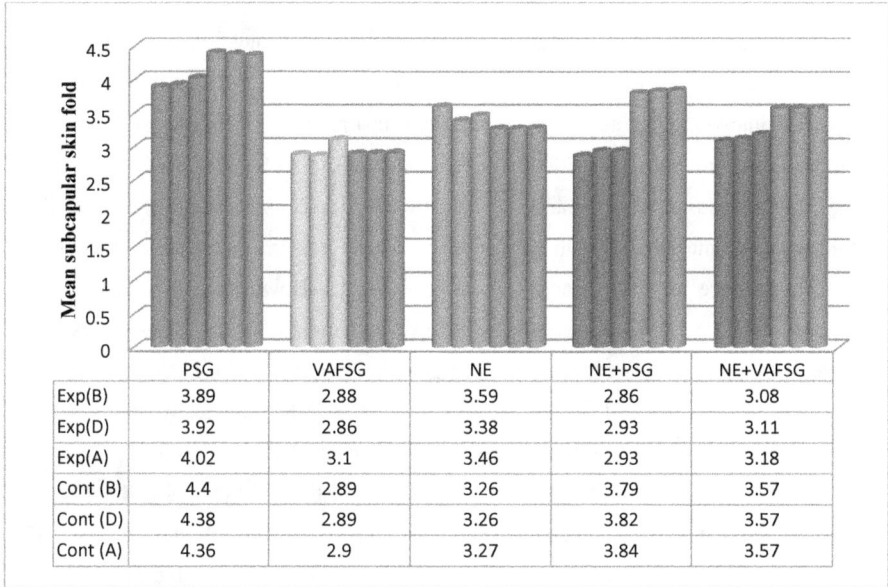

	PSG	VAFSG	NE	NE+PSG	NE+VAFSG
Exp(B)	3.89	2.88	3.59	2.86	3.08
Exp(D)	3.92	2.86	3.38	2.93	3.11
Exp(A)	4.02	3.1	3.46	2.93	3.18
Cont (B)	4.4	2.89	3.26	3.79	3.57
Cont (D)	4.38	2.89	3.26	3.82	3.57
Cont (A)	4.36	2.9	3.27	3.84	3.57

**Fig. 4.43 Per cent change in Sabcapular Skinfold Thickness of the pre-school
children before   during and after interventions**

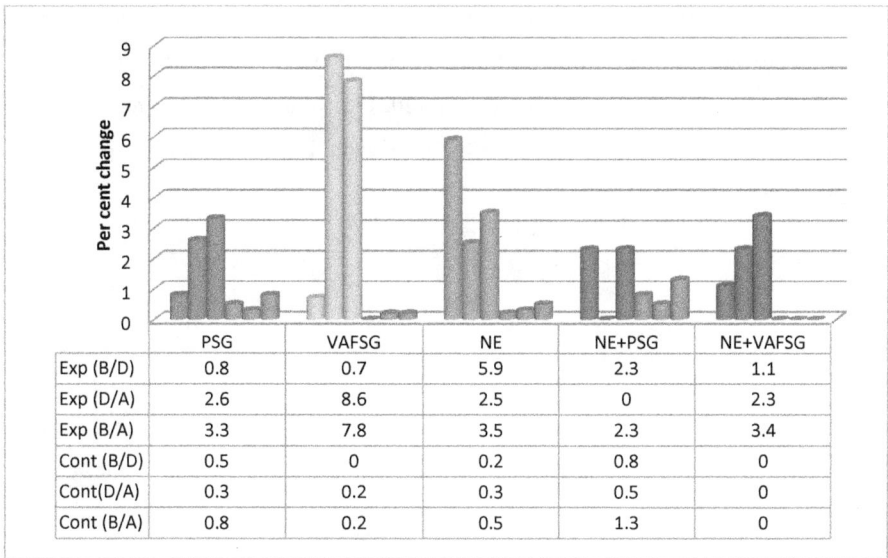

	PSG	VAFSG	NE	NE+PSG	NE+VAFSG
Exp (B/D)	0.8	0.7	5.9	2.3	1.1
Exp (D/A)	2.6	8.6	2.5	0	2.3
Exp (B/A)	3.3	7.8	3.5	2.3	3.4
Cont (B/D)	0.5	0	0.2	0.8	0
Cont(D/A)	0.3	0.2	0.3	0.5	0
Cont (B/A)	0.8	0.2	0.5	1.3	0

4.5.8 Efficacy of nutrition interventions on Triceps Skinfold Thickness of the pre-school children

In continuation to the measurement of subscapular skin fold thickness, the experiment was also carried out to measure triceps skin fold thickness for the efficacy of the nutrition interventions, and the measurement (mm) for the control and experimental group spread over five nutrition interventions PSG, VAFSG, NE, NE+PSG, and NE+VAFSG presented in the table 4.17. It is clear from the table that the triceps skin fold thickness measurements in respect of the control sub-groups for all interventions did not produce any significant changes at all stages. However, experimental sub-groups of PSG, VAFSG, and NE+VAFSG have shown some impact as per analysis in table 4.17. Among PSG experimental sub-group 6 per cent and 6.2 per cent change was observed at D/A and B/A, and the same was found to be statistically significant at $p \leq 0.01$. For VAFSG experimental group, 2.1 per cent, 2 per cent and 4.1 per cent mean change at all the three stages was also found to be statistically significant at 5 per cent and 1 per cent, respectively. Findings of present study indicates existence of visual impact of VAFSG on the triceps in the study area at all the stages of measurements. NE+VAFSG experiment sub-group also represented 9 per cent and 7.2 per cent mean change at D/A and B/A which were significant ($p \leq 0.01$) statistically.

On the basis of the above analysis, the researcher is of the view that PSG and VAFSG may contribute to the growth of the triceps in the long run as in subscapular skinfold thickness. On contrary, López-Alonso *et.al,* (2021) also reported that paired analysis showed high increment of anthropometric parameters in the experimental group as compared to control group.

Table: 4.17 Efficacy of nutrition interventions on the Triceps Skin fold Thickness of the pre-school children during different stages of interventions

Experimental Groups		Actual Increase			Mean change								t value		
		Before (0day)	During (60days)	After (120days)	B/D		D/A		B/A				B/D (0-60 days)	D/A (60-120 days)	B/A (0-120 days)
					Total	%	Total	%	Total	%					
PSG	Control	2.64±0.68	2.63±0.76	2.76±0.62	0.01	0.3	0.13	4.8	0.12	4.5			0.090	1.700	1.710
	Experimental	2.58±0.21	2.28±0.21	2.74±0.24	0.01	0.2	0.15	6	0.16	6.2			1	2.97**	3.04**
VAFSG	Control	2.80±0.33	2.81±0.31	2.81±0.32	0.02	0.5	0.01	0.2	0.01	0.4			1.37	1	0.8
	Experimental	2.90±0.45	2.96±0.44	3.02±0.42	0.06	2.1	0.06	2	0.12	4.1			2.10*	2.85**	3.09**
N.E	Control	2.42±0.21	2.43±0.19	2.48±0.19	0.01	0.4	0.05	2.1	0.06	2.5			0.52	1.19	1.13
	Experimental	2.37±0.34	2.37±0.34	2.47±0.17	0	0	0.1	4.2	0.1	4.2			0	1.35	1.35
NE+PSG	Control	2.54±0.20	2.54±0.19	2.51±0.17	0	0	0.03	1.4	0.03	1.4			0	1.45	1.16
	Experimental	2.47±0.28	2.52±0.28	2.52±0.28	0.05	2	0	0	0.05	2			0.7	0	0.7
NE+VAFSG	Control	2.72±0.47	2.72±0.47	2.73±0.47	0	0.2	0.01	0.2	0.01	0.4			1	0.56	1
	Experimental	2.44±0.48	2.40±0.49	2.61±0.45	0.04	1.6	0.22	9	0.18	7.2			0.66	3.56**	2.04

**significant at p≤0.01, *significant at p≤ 0.05

CONTROL– No Intervention

PSG- Probiotic supplemented group; VAFSG –Value-added food supplemented group; NE –Nutrition education; NE+PSG- Nutrition education+ Probiotic supplemented group; NE +VAFSG – Nutrition education + value -added food supplemented group

B/D – Before / During D/A- During/ After B/A– Before/ After

111

Fig. 4.44 Mean Triecep Skinfold Thickness of pre-school children during different stages of nutrition interventions

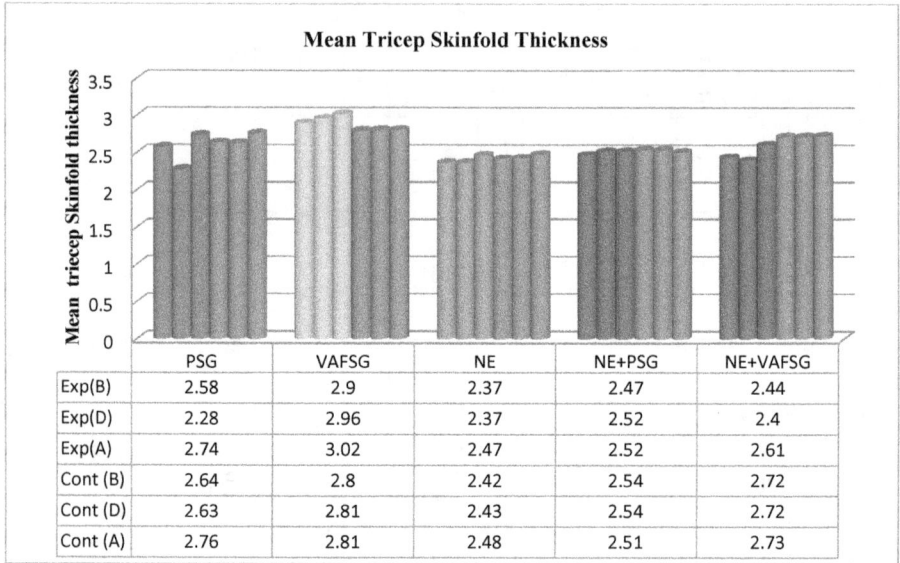

Mean Tricep Skinfold Thickness

	PSG	VAFSG	NE	NE+PSG	NE+VAFSG
Exp(B)	2.58	2.9	2.37	2.47	2.44
Exp(D)	2.28	2.96	2.37	2.52	2.4
Exp(A)	2.74	3.02	2.47	2.52	2.61
Cont (B)	2.64	2.8	2.42	2.54	2.72
Cont (D)	2.63	2.81	2.43	2.54	2.72
Cont (A)	2.76	2.81	2.48	2.51	2.73

Fig. 4.45 Per cent change in Triceps Skinfold Thickness of the pre-school children before during and after intervention

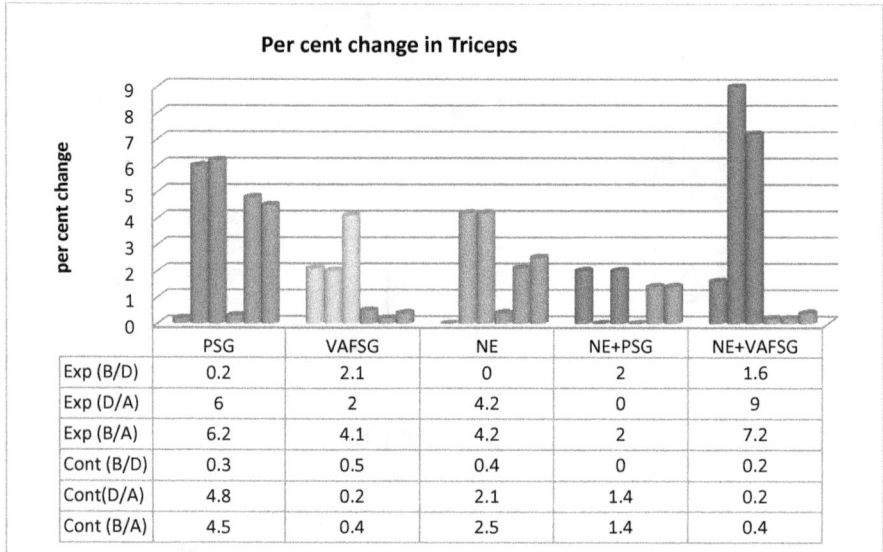

Per cent change in Triceps

	PSG	VAFSG	NE	NE+PSG	NE+VAFSG
Exp (B/D)	0.2	2.1	0	2	1.6
Exp (D/A)	6	2	4.2	0	9
Exp (B/A)	6.2	4.1	4.2	2	7.2
Cont (B/D)	0.3	0.5	0.4	0	0.2
Cont(D/A)	4.8	0.2	2.1	1.4	0.2
Cont (B/A)	4.5	0.4	2.5	1.4	0.4

4.5.9 Efficacy of nutrition interventions on Total Protein of the pre-school children

PSG: Mean total protein values for subgroups of experimental and control of probiotic supplemented group were 6.33±0.41g/dl,6.35±0.45g/dl, 6.51±0.42g/d and 6.04±0.81g/dl,5.99±0.82, 6.16±0.75g/dl before, during and after studied period, respectively. In experimental sub-group gradual increase (0.3-2.8%) in total protein was observed during the whole duration of studied period, whereas in control sub-group maximum improvement was noticed at 60-120 days (during the study). Statistically analysis further expressed non-significant change among both the sub-groups. Hence it could be concluded that PSG is not contributing for much increase in the protein values in the study area.

VAFSG: For value added food supplemented experimental sub-group, the mean values of total protein at zero, 60 days and 120 days were 6.22±0.51g/dl, 6.37±0.31g/dl and 6.51±0.27g/dl, respectively. An increase in mean percentage as 2.5, 2.2 and 4.7 per cent was noticed as compared to almost nil improvement among corresponding control sub-group. Highly significant ($p \leq 0.05$ & $p \leq 0.01$) increment at all three phases of the experimental trial confirmed good impact of VAFSG on the total protein content as per analysis.

NE: Nutrition education experimental sub groups presented little improvement of only 0.7 per cent in mean per cent of total protein. Hence, no significant changes were observed in both the sub-groups of nutrition education group. Control sub-group showed gradual improvement from 0.1 to 0.3 per cent during the whole study period but statistically the increment was non-significant.

NE+PSG: Mean total protein values for experimental group were 6.10±0.37g/ dl,6.33±0.45g/dl and 6.35±0.48g/dl at before, during and after experimental trial, respectively. Experimental sub-group, showed significant changes ($p \leq 0.01$) of 3.8 and 4.1 per cent respectively after 60 and 120 days of intervention. On the contrary control subgroup to whom no intervention was provided showed very negligible per cent changes of 0.3 & 0.03 during the study period. It could be inferred that NE+PSG can be referred as a good trial.

NE+VAFSG: Mean respective total protein values of the experimental sub-group were 6.03±0.43g/dl, 6.10±0.35g/dl and 6.35±0.30g/dl at 0, 60 and 120 days of experimental trial. A steady improvement in mean percentage of 1.2, 4.1 and 5.4 per

113

Table: 4.18 Efficacy of nutrition interventions on the Total Protein of the pre-school children during different stages of interventions

Nutrition Interventions		Actual Increase			Mean change						t value		
		Before (0day)	During (60days)	After (120days)	B/D		D/A		B/A		B/D (0day)	D/A (60-120 days)	B/A (0-120 days)
					Total	%	Total	%	Total	%			
PSG	Control	6.04±0.81	5.99±0.82	6.16±0.75	0.06	0.9	0.17	2.8	0.12	1.9	1.44	2.07	1.41
	Experimental	6.33±0.41	6.35±0.45	6.51±0.42	0.02	0.3	0.16	2.5	0.18	2.8	1	2.07	2.07
VAFSG	Control	5.98±0.30	5.98±0.29	5.98±0.26	0	0.1	0	0.1	0	0	0.56	0.43	0
	Experimental	6.22±0.51	6.37±0.31	6.51±0.27	0.15	2.5	0.14	2.2	0.3	4.7	2.54*	2.64*	3.49**
N.E	Control	5.87±0.31	5.88±0.29	5.89±0.32	0	0.1	0.01	0.2	0.01	0.3	0.56	0.69	0.9
	Experimental	5.97±0.32	5.97±0.32	6.01±0.36	0	0	0.04	0.7	0.04	0.7	0	1.28	1.28
N.E+PSG	Control	5.94±0.19	5.92±0.17	5.92±0.17	0.01	0.3	0	0	0.01	0.03	0.9	0	0.82
	Experimental	6.10±0.37	6.33±0.45	6.35±0.48	0.23	3.8	0.02	0.3	0.25	4.1	3.89**	0.8	4.50**
N.E+ VAFSG	Control	5.88±0.26	5.87±0.26	5.87±0.27	0	0.1	0	0.1	0.01	0.2	1	1	1.45
	Experimental	6.03±0.43	6.10±0.35	6.35±0.30	0.07	1.2	0.25	4.1	0.32	5.4	2.54*	3.11**	3.72**

***significant at p≤0.01, *significant at p≤ 0.05

CONTROL– No Intervention

PSG- Probiotic supplemented group; VAFSG –Value-added food supplemented group; NE –Nutrition education; NE+PSG- Nutrition education+ Probiotic supplemented group; NE +VAFSG – Nutrition education + value -added food supplemented group

B/D – Before / During D/A- During/ After B/A– Before/ After

114

cent was reported during the different phases of trial among experimental sub-group. Statistically highly significant ($p \leq 0.01$) increment was observed at all the stages of experimental trial of four months. Control subgroup subjects didn't show any improvement in their total protein values. Almost negligible improvement in total protein values among control subgroup confirmed efficacy of NE+VAFSG on total values.

Comparatively, mean per cent change was found to be highest among N.E + VAFSG (5.4%), followed by VAFSG (4.7%), NE+PSG and PSG (4.1%). It can be safely concluded that NE+VAFSG and VAFSG experimental sub-groups represented significant difference for B/D ($p \leq 0.05$), D/A ($p \leq 0.05$), and B/A ($p \leq 0.01$). Further it confirmed the efficacy of these interventions on total protein improvement. For NE +PSG experimental group B/D and B/A have shown a good impact ($p \leq 0.01$). It is interesting to note that NE did not show any impact on total protein. Further, majority of the values of t static were non-significant except experimental sub-groups of NE+ VAFSG, VAFSG and NE +PSG which have shown significant improvement ($p \leq 0.05$ and $p \leq 0.01$) as evident in the above table 4.18.

Table 4.19 Analysis of Variance for Total Protein before, during and after nutrition intervention

	Before					During					After				
	SS	DF	MS	F	P	SS	DF	MS	F	P	SS	DF	MS	F	P
Between Groups	1.655	4	0.414			2.542	4	0.635			3.302	4	0.826		
Within Groups	16.583	95	0.175	2.37	0.058	14.236	95	0.15	4.24	0.003	13.626	95	0.143	5.756	<0.001
Total	18.237	99				16.777	99				16.928	99			

Statistically analysis (ANOVA) further indicated a significant ($p < 0.01$) improvement of total protein among all experimental sub-groups subjects after 120 days of complete interventions. Inferences made through Tukey Multiple Comparison test revealed a significant ($p < 0.01$) difference in the mean values in mid (0-60day) of experimental in between PSG and NE, NE+VAFSG ,in between VAFSG and NE, NE+VAFSG and in between NE and NE+PSG respectively. While During/After (60-120days) significant ($p < 0.01$) improvement was observed in between PSG and NE, NE+VAFSG and in between VAFSG and NE, in between NE and NE+PSG. After 120 days Tukey post hoc test divulged highly significant (($p < 0.00$) improvement in

between PSG & NE and VAFSG & NE respectively. Nutrition education experimental group also showed significant (p< 0.01) increment in between NE+PSG and NE +VAFSG.

Fig. 4.46 Mean Total Protein of pre-school children during different stages of interventions

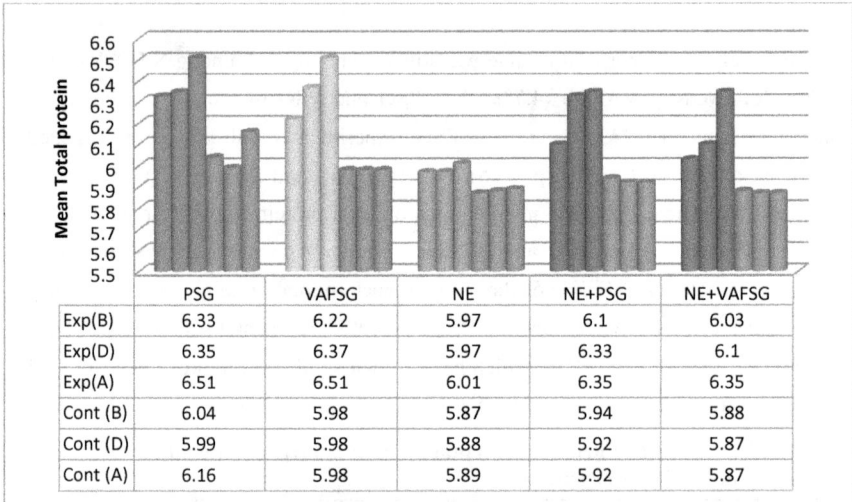

	PSG	VAFSG	NE	NE+PSG	NE+VAFSG
Exp(B)	6.33	6.22	5.97	6.1	6.03
Exp(D)	6.35	6.37	5.97	6.33	6.1
Exp(A)	6.51	6.51	6.01	6.35	6.35
Cont (B)	6.04	5.98	5.87	5.94	5.88
Cont (D)	5.99	5.98	5.88	5.92	5.87
Cont (A)	6.16	5.98	5.89	5.92	5.87

Fig. 4.47 Per cent change in Total protein in pre-school children before, during and after intervention

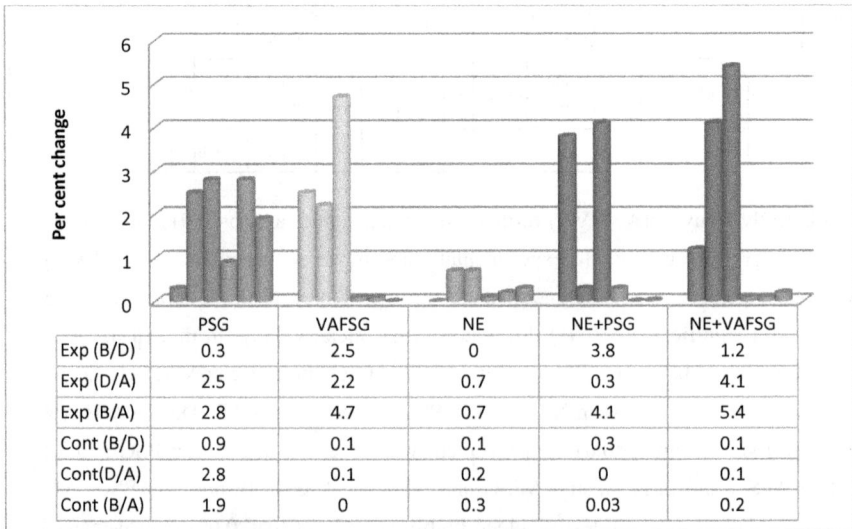

	PSG	VAFSG	NE	NE+PSG	NE+VAFSG
Exp (B/D)	0.3	2.5	0	3.8	1.2
Exp (D/A)	2.5	2.2	0.7	0.3	4.1
Exp (B/A)	2.8	4.7	0.7	4.1	5.4
Cont (B/D)	0.9	0.1	0.1	0.3	0.1
Cont(D/A)	2.8	0.1	0.2	0	0.1
Cont (B/A)	1.9	0	0.3	0.03	0.2

Table 4.20 Multiple Comparisons for Total protein of pre-school children before, during and after nutrition interventions Tukey HSD

Dependent Variable			Mean Difference (I-J)	Std. Error	P Value
Total Protein Before	PSG	VAFSG	0.11	0.13	0.92
		NE	0.36	0.13	0.06
		NE+PSG	0.23	0.13	0.44
		NE+VAFSG	0.3	0.13	0.16
	VAFSG	NE	0.25	0.13	0.35
		NE+PSG	0.12	0.13	0.91
		NE+VAFSG	0.19	0.13	0.6
	NE	NE+PSG	-0.13	0.13	0.86
		NE+VAFSG	-0.06	0.13	0.99
	NE+PSG	NE+VAFSG	0.07	0.13	0.98
Total Protein During	PSG	VAFSG	-0.03	0.12	1
		NE	.37500*	0.12	0.02
		NE+PSG	0.01	0.12	1
		NE+VAFSG	0.24	0.12	0.27
	VAFSG	NE	.40*	0.12	0.01
		NE+PSG	0.04	0.12	1
		NE+VAFSG	0.27	0.12	0.19
	NE	NE+PSG	-.36*	0.12	0.03
		NE+VAFSG	-0.13	0.12	0.83
	NE+PSG	NE+PSG	0.23	0.12	0.34
Total Protein After	PSG	VAFSG	0	0.12	1
		NE	.49500*	0.12	0
		NE+PSG	0.16	0.12	0.7
		NE+VAFSG	0.16	0.12	0.7
	VAFSG	NE	.50*	0.12	0
		NE+PSG	0.16	0.12	0.67
		NE+VAFSG	0.16	0.12	0.67
	NE	NE+PSG	-.34*	0.12	0.04
		NE+VAFSG	-.34*	0.12	0.04
	NE+PSG	NE+VAFSG	0	0.12	1

Table: 4.21 Efficacy of nutrition interventions on the Serum Albumin of the pre-school children during different stages of interventions

Nutrition Interventions		Actual Increase			Mean change						t value		
		Before (0days)	During (60days)	After (120days)	B/D		D/A		B/A		B/D (0-60days)	D/A (60-120days)	B/A (0-120days)
					Total	%	Total	%	Total	%			
PSG	Control	3.41±0.64	3.31±0.70	3.43±0.59	0.1	2.9	0.12	3.6	0.02	0.6	0.870	1.010	0.650
	Experimental	3.79±0.45	3.79±0.50	3.81±0.49	0.01	0.1	0.02	0.4	0.02	0.5	0.17	0.24	0.29
VAFSG	Control	2.95±0.41	2.96±0.41	2.96±0.41	0	0.2	0.01	0.2	0.01	0.3	1	0.56	1
	Experimental	3.64±0.60	3.81±0.54	3.89±0.52	0.17	4.8	0.07	2	0.25	6.9	3.38**	2.51*	4.94**
N.E	Control	3±0.24	3±0.23	3±0.23	0	0.2	0	0.2	0	0	0.56	0.56	0
	Experimental	2.84±0.55	2.84±0.58	2.85±0.95	0	0.2	0.01	0.4	0.02	0.5	0.11	0.07	0.1
N.E+PSG	Control	3.14±0.37	3.12±0.36	3.14±0.36	0.02	0.6	0.02	0.5	0	0.2	1.45	1.37	0.27
	Experimental	3.38±0.35	3.55±0.36	3.83±0.28	0.17	5	0.28	7.9	0.45	13.3	2.76*	4.41**	5.74**
N.E+VAFSG	Control	2.69±0.46	2.70±0.45	2.69±0.43	0.02	0.6	0.01	0.4	0	0.2	1	0.8	0.37
	Experimental	3.29±0.47	3.49±0.45	3.69±0.51	0.2	6.1	0.21	5.9	0.41	12.3	5.21**	2.90**	5.36**

**significant at p≤0.01, *significant at p≤0.05

CONTROL– No Intervention

PSG- Probiotic supplemented group; VAFSG –Value added food supplemented group; N.E –Nutrition education; N.E+PSG- Nutrition education+ Probiotic supplemented group; N.E +VAFSG – Nutrition education + value added food supplemented group

B/D – Before / During D/A- During/ After B/A– Before/ After

4.5.10 Efficacy of nutrition intervention on Serum albumin of the pre-school children

PSG: The data generated through experiment on serum albumin was analysed statistically and presented in table 4.21. In the experimental sub-group the mean serum albumin values were 3.79±0.45g/dl, 3.79±0.50g/dl, and 3.81±0.49g/dl on before, during, and after studied period, respectively. Respective average serum albumin of control sub-group were 3.41±0.64g/dl, 3.31±0.70g/dl, and 3.43±0.59g/dl. The effect of probiotic supplementation was almost non existence in experimental group as evident in the analysis. However improved mean percentage of 2.9 and 3.6 per cent among control sub-group was noticed which further reduced to only 0.6 per cent at the end of study which could be due to some sample error or other natural factors.

VAFSG: The observed mean serum albumin values in the experimental group at 0, 60 and 120 days were 3.64±0.60g/dl, 3.81±0.54g/dl and 3.89±0.52g/dl respectively .For control group there seems to be no changes up to the completion to the study. Feeding intervention showed improvement of 6.9 per cent after 120 days, 4.8 per cent for 60 days and 2 per cent for D/A (60-120days) and these mean differences have also been observed significantly ($p \leq 0.01$ and $p \leq 0.05$) different on compared use of paired t-test. On the contrary control sub-group didn't show any change in their respective serum albumin values during the complete study period.

NE: The mean values of serum albumin of the experimental and control sub-group remained same throughout the whole studied period i.e. 2.84±0.55g/dl, 2.84±0.58, and 2.85±0.95 and 3±0.24g/dl, 3±0.23g/dl, and 3±0.23g/dl, respectively. As per analysis controls as well as experimental group both were not showing any impact of nutrition education on the serum albumin parameters.

NE+PSG: In respect of serum albumin content in the blood sample, NE+PSG intervention has shown good impact among the experimental sub-group subjects, as evident by the mean values i.e. 3.38±0.35g/dl, 3.55±0.36g/dl and 3.83±0.28g/dl at before, during and after trial period, respectively. Whereas no change was found in control sub-group subjects. Further analysis showed mean per cent change of 13.3 (B/A), 7.9 (D/A) and 5.0 (B/D) in the experimental subjects which was highest amongst all the other intervention sub-groups. Furthermore, statistically significant (p≤0.01) values at all the three stages of intervention period proved efficacy of combined nutrition education and probiotic supplementation on improvement serum albumin values. On the other hand control sub-group subjects present only negligible change/improvement during the whole study period.

NE+VAFSG: It is clear from the data that in the control sub-group respondents, there was almost negligible change in mean serum albumin values. During the different stages of intervention, the mean serum albumin values of experimental sub-group of NE+VAFSG were 3.29±0.47g/dl,3.49±0.45g/dl and 3.69±0.51g/dl. A good percentage change of 12.3 per cent (B/A), 6.1 per cent (B/D) and 5.9 per cent in D/A of experimental sub-group represented quiet significant (p≤0.01) effect as tested statistically.

The highest mean change was observed for B/A (13.3%) in N.E +PSG treatment group in the experimental sample followed by 12.3 per cent in B/A for experimental sample of NE +VAFSG and 6.9 per cent in B/A of VAFSG experimental subjects. Most of the t values for serum albumin effect in rest of sub-groups were non-significant. It indicates that for both control as well as experimental sub-groups mean scores showing some variations may be attributed to sampling fluctuations as the groups were little bit at variant due to age, gender, height and weight etc, and may not affect the conduct of experiment. As a sum-up of the experiment it could be further pointed out that VAFSG, NE+PSG, and NE+VAFSG are standing in a same row. In other words, all these nutrition interventions can be thought to be equally affected on the experiment as per analysis in table 4.21. The study indicated that pattern of response is almost the same as that of total protein (table 4.18) except that D/A was also showing a good impact of NE +PSG in experimental subgroups. The study indicated that NE+ PSG has shown maximum efficacy of nutrition intervention in the estimation of serum albumin on the sample in the study area. For paired t-values VAFSG, NE+ VAFSG are showing similar trend for respective intervention on the serum albumin content in the blood sample in the study area.

Table 4.22 Analysis of Variance for Serum Albumin before during and after intervention

	Before					During					After				
	SS	DF	MS	F	P	SS	DF	MS	F	P	SS	DF	MS	F	P
Between Groups	10.702	4	2.675			12.357	4	3.089			14.877	4	3.719		
Within Groups	23.5	95	0.247	10.816	<0.001	23.359	95	0.246	12.564	<0.001	33.901	95	0.357	10.423	<0.001
Total	34.201	99				35.716	99				48.778	99			

ANOVA (analysis of variance) for Serum albumin results revealed highly significant ($p< 0.01$) improvement among all the experimental sub-groups on various nutrition interventions for 120 days. Ensuing of data reflected that the mean albumin through Tukey multiple comparison test was highly significantly ($p< 0.01$) in between PSG and NE, NE+VAFSG, in between VAFSG and NE, NE+VAFSG and in between NE and NE+PSG, NE+VAFSG in mid (0-60days) of intervention trial. While during (60-120days) the nutrition intervention highly significant difference ($p< 0.00$) in serum albumin values appeared in between PSG and NE, NE+PSG, in between VAFSG and NE, in between NE and NE+PSG, in between NE and NE+VAFSG. After 120days a highly significant difference ($p<0.00$) was found in between PSG and NE, in between VAFSG and NE, in between NE and NE+PSG, NE+VAFSG respectively

121

Fig. 4.48 Mean Serum Albumin in children during different stages of interventions

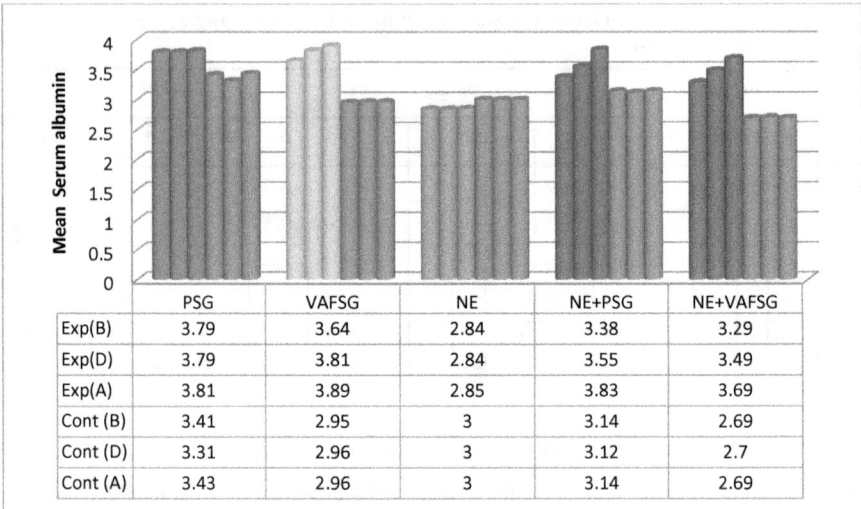

	PSG	VAFSG	NE	NE+PSG	NE+VAFSG
Exp(B)	3.79	3.64	2.84	3.38	3.29
Exp(D)	3.79	3.81	2.84	3.55	3.49
Exp(A)	3.81	3.89	2.85	3.83	3.69
Cont (B)	3.41	2.95	3	3.14	2.69
Cont (D)	3.31	2.96	3	3.12	2.7
Cont (A)	3.43	2.96	3	3.14	2.69

Fig. 4.49 Per cent change in Serum Albumin in pre-school children before, during and after intervention

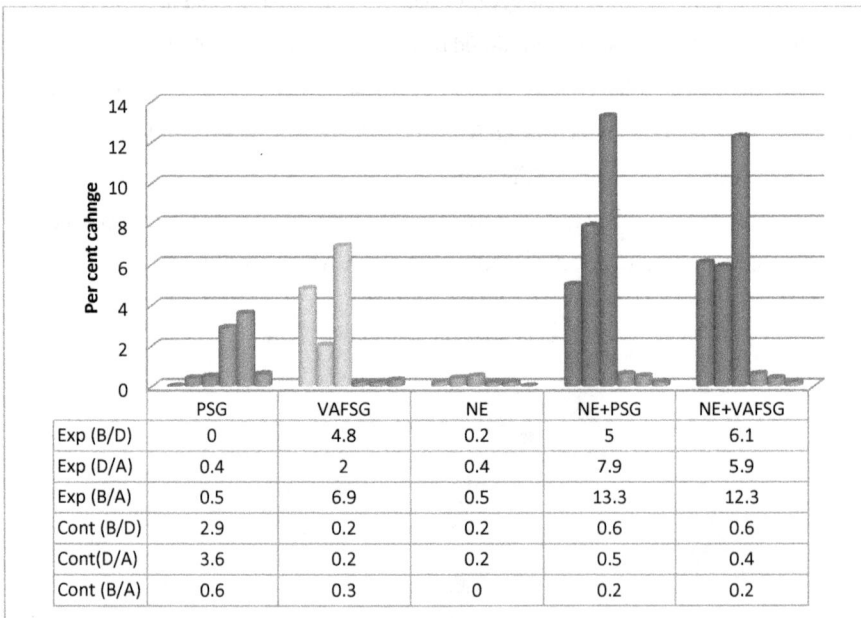

	PSG	VAFSG	NE	NE+PSG	NE+VAFSG
Exp (B/D)	0	4.8	0.2	5	6.1
Exp (D/A)	0.4	2	0.4	7.9	5.9
Exp (B/A)	0.5	6.9	0.5	13.3	12.3
Cont (B/D)	2.9	0.2	0.2	0.6	0.6
Cont(D/A)	3.6	0.2	0.2	0.5	0.4
Cont (B/A)	0.6	0.3	0	0.2	0.2

Table 4.23 Multiple Comparisons for Serum Albumin of pre-school children before, during and after nutrition interventions Tukey HSD

Dependent Variable			Mean Difference (I-J)	Std. Error	P Value
Serum Albumin Before	PSG	VAFSG	0.15	0.16	0.87
		NE	.95*	0.16	0
		NE+PSG	0.41	0.16	0.08
		NE+VAFSG	.50*	0.16	0.02
	VAFSG	NE	.80*	0.16	0
		NE+PSG	0.26	0.16	0.47
		NE+VAFSG	0.35	0.16	0.18
	NE	NE+PSG	-.54*	0.16	0.01
		NE+VAFSG	-.45*	0.16	0.04
	NE+PSG	NE+VAFSG	0.09	0.16	0.98
Serum Albumin During	PSG	VAFSG	-0.02	0.16	1
		NE	.95*	0.16	0
		NE+PSG	0.25	0.16	0.53
		NE+VAFSG	0.31	0.16	0.3
	VAFSG	NE	.97*	0.16	0
		NE+PSG	0.27	0.16	0.45
		NE+VAFSG	0.33	0.16	0.24
	NE	NE+PSG	-.70500*	0.16	0
		NE+VAFSG	-.64500*	0.16	0
	NE+PSG	NE+VAFSG	0.06	0.16	1
Serum Albumin After	PSG	VAFSG	-0.08	0.19	0.99
		NE	.95500*	0.19	0
		NE+PSG	-0.02	0.19	1
		NE+VAFSG	0.12	0.19	0.97
	VAFSG	NE	1.03500*	0.19	0
		NE+PSG	0.06	0.19	1
		NE+VAFSG	0.19	0.19	0.84
	NE	NE+PSG	-.97500*	0.19	0
		NE+VAFSG	-.84*	0.19	0
	NE+PSG	NE+VAFSG	0.14	0.19	0.95

Table: 4.24 Efficacy of nutrition interventions on the Serum Globulin of the pre-school children during different stages of interventions

Nutrition Interventions		Actual Increase			Mean change						t value		
		Before (0 day)	During (60 days)	After (120 days)	B/D		D/A		B/A		B/D (0-60 days)	D/A (60-120 days)	B/A (0-120 days)
					Total	%	Total	%	Total	%			
PSG	Control	2.63±0.78	2.68±0.89	2.73±0.66	0.05	1.7	0.05	1.9	0.1	3.6	0.470	0.380	1.130
	Experimental	2.54±0.64	2.56±0.69	2.70±0.64	0.02	0.6	0.15	5.7	0.16	6.3	0.42	1.34	1.57
VAFSG	Control	3.03±0.37	3.03±0.37	3.02±0.36	0	0	0.01	0.3	0.01	0.3	0	0.69	0.52
	Experimental	2.58±0.59	2.56±0.59	2.63±0.50	0.02	0.8	0.06	2.5	0.04	1.7	0.28	1.04	0.49
N.E	Control	2.87±0.24	2.88±0.23	2.89±0.25	0.01	0.3	0.01	0.2	0.02	0.5	0.8	0.29	0.67
	Experimental	3.14±0.52	3.13±0.58	3.16±0.94	0.01	0.2	0.03	1	0.02	0.8	0.11	0.22	0.17
N.E+PSG	Control	2.80±0.42	2.80±0.40	2.80±0.40	0.01	0.2	0.02	0.5	0.01	0.04	0.22	1.14	0.04
	Experimental	2.73±0.49	2.79±0.58	2.53±0.52	0.06	2.2	0.26	9.3	0.2	7.3	0.72	4.18**	2.28*
N.E+ VAFSG	Control	3.19±0.55	3.17±0.53	3.18±0.53	0.02	0.6	0.01	0.2	0.01	0.5	1.28	0.37	1
	Experimental	2.74±0.64	2.62±0.59	2.66±0.65	0.13	4.6	0.05	1.7	0.08	2.9	2.54*	0.4	0.71

**significant at p≤0.01, *significant at p≤ 0.05

CONTROL– No Intervention

-PSG- Probiotic supplemented group; VAFSG –Value-added food supplemented group; NE –Nutrition education; NE+PSG- Nutrition education+ Probiotic supplemented group; NE +VAFSG – Nutrition education + value -added food supplemented group

B/D – Before / During D/A- During/ After B/A– Before/ After

4.5.11 Efficacy of nutrition interventions on Serum Globulin of the pre-school children

PSG: The mean serum globulin values of the experimental and control sub-groups were 2.54±0.64g/dl, 2.56±0.69g/dl, 2.70±0.64g/dl and 2.63±0.78g/dl, 2.68±0.89g/dl,2.73±0.66g/dl at 0 days, 60 days and 120 days, respectively. Gradual improvement from 0.6-6.3 per cent among experimental and from 1.7 to 3.6 per cent among control subjects values was noticed. Comparatively, much more per cent increase in serum globulin was reported in experimental sub-group with 6.3 per cent improvement as compared to only 3.6 per cent among control sub-groups at the end of the study period. Probiotic supplemented group showed maximum improvement of 6.3 per cent at the end of the study (120 days) but the improvement was non- significant statistically.

VAFSG: The observed mean values in the experimental sub-group were 2.58±0.59g/dl, 2.56±0.59g/dl, and 2.63±0.50g/dl during different stages of intervention and almost similar trend (3.03±0.37g/dl, 3.03±0.37g/dl, 3.02±0.36g/dl) was found in control sub-group. No significant impact was seen in studied period as mean percentage changes in control sub-group was almost of zero order and a change of 2.5 per cent for B/D in the experimental sub-group was noticed.

NE: The mean serum globulin values in the experimental sub-group were 3.14±0.52g/dl, 3.13±0.58g/dl and 3.16±0.94g/dl at before, during, and after nutrition education intervention, respectively. The observed respective mean values of the control group were 2.87±0.24g/dl, 2.88±0.23g/dl, and 2.89±0.25g/dl. The mean percentage change was negligible (0.8 and 0.5) in both the respective sub-groups hence; no significant increment was reported in the nutrition education intervention trial. Further analysis of the data revealed that the impact of nutrition education intervention was of the same pattern as that of PSG and VAFSG as is evident in table 4.24 and cannot be taken as significant effect on mean serum globulin levels in the study area.

NE+PSG: The mean values of serum globulin in the experimental and control sub-groups were 2.73±0.49g/dl, 2.79±0.58g/dl,2.53±0.52g/dl and 2.80±0.42g/dl, 2.80±0.40g/dl, 2.80±0.40g/dl at starting, mid and completion of the intervention trial period, respectively. In control sub-group, there was effect of almost zero-order however in the experimental sub-group mean per cent change of 9.3 per cent was observed for D/A (60-120days) and 7.3 per cent for B/A (0-120days) which were significantly different at 1 per cent and 5 per cent, respectively. Thus, NE+PSG

125

intervention trial was significantly (p≤0.01) effective in improving the serum globulin level during the experimentation at the stages of D/A and B/A but not at B/D.

NE+VAFSG: The data collected showed mean serum globulin value of the experimental sub-group as 2.74±0.64g/dl, 2.62±0.59g/dl, and 2.66±0.65g/dl at different stages of intervention trial. The respective average values of the control sub-group were 3.19±0.55g/dl,3.17±0.53g/dl, and 3.18±0.53. The control sub-group reported no specific trend, however experimental sub-group have shown a maximum percentage change of 4.6 at the starting (B/D) with t value significant at 5 per cent.

The comparative analysis table 4.24 indicated a maximum mean per cent change of 9.3 in the case of the experimental sub-group intervened with nutrition education along with probiotic supplementation. The perusal of the data further indicated that according to paired t-test applied, the t static for D/A (p≤0.01), B/A in the experimental sample of NE +PSG (p≤0.05), and only B/D in the experimental sample of NE+VAFSG (p≤0.05) were showing the significant impact of nutrition interventions on serum globulin levels of respective subjects.

Table 4.25 Analysis of Variance for Serum Globulin Before During and After intervention

	Before					During						After					
	SS	DF	MS	F	P	SS	DF	MS	F	P	SS	DF	MS	F	P	SS	DF
Between Groups	4.435	4	1.109			4.715	4	1.179				Between Groups 4.873	4	1.218			
Within Groups	32.451	95	0.342	3.246	0.015	35.391	95	0.373	3.164	0.017		Within Groups 43.031	95	0.453		2.69	0.036
Total	36.886	99				40.106	99					Total 47.904	99				

Statistically analysis (ANOVA) indicated significant (p<0.01) improvement of serum globulin in all experimental sub-groups subjects after 120 days of complete interventions. On further examination of the data, by Tukey multiple comparison test results indicated a highly significant improvement (p<0.00) in serum globulin in between PSG and NE, in between VAFSG and NE, in between NE and NE+PSG after 0-60 days. While during (60-120 days) the intervention trial significant difference was observed in between PSG and NE, in between VAFSG and NE, in between NE and NE+VAFSG, in between NE+PSG and NE+VAFSG. Further analysis after 120 days of nutrition intervention trial showed significant difference (p< 0.01) in between PSG and NE, in between VAFSG and NE, in between NE and NE+PSG, NE+VAFSG.

Table 4.26 Multiple Comparisons for Serum Globulin of pre-school children before, during and after nutrition interventions Tukey HSD

Dependent Variable			Mean Difference (I-J)	Std. Error	P Value
Serum Globulin Before	PSG	VAFSG	-0.04	0.18	1
		NE	-.59500*	0.18	0.01
		NE+PSG	-0.19	0.18	0.85
		NE+VAFSG	-0.2	0.18	0.82
	VAFSG	NE	-.55500*	0.18	0.03
		NE+PSG	-0.15	0.18	0.93
		NE_VAFSG	-0.16	0.18	0.91
	NE	NE+PSG	0.41	0.18	0.18
		NE+VAFSG	0.4	0.18	0.21
	NE+PSG	NE+VAFSG	-0.02	0.18	1
Serum Globulin During	PSG	VAFSG	0	0.19	1
		NE	-.57500*	0.19	0.03
		NE+PSG	-0.23	0.19	0.76
		NE+VAFSG	-0.06	0.19	1
	VAFSG	NE	-.57*	0.19	0.03
		NE+PSG	-0.23	0.19	0.77
		NE+VAFSG	-0.05	0.19	1
	NE	NE+PSG	0.35	0.19	0.39
		NE+VAFSG	0.52	0.19	0.07
	NE+PSG	NE+VAFSG	0.17	0.19	0.9
Serum Globulin After	PSG	VAFSG	0.08	0.21	1
		NE	-0.46	0.21	0.2
		NE+PSG	0.18	0.21	0.92
		NE+VAFSG	0.04	0.21	1
	VAFSG	NE	-0.54	0.21	0.1
		NE+PSG	0.1	0.21	0.99
		NE+VAFSG	-0.04	0.21	1
	NE	NE+PSG	.63500*	0.21	0.03
		NE+VAFSG	0.5	0.21	0.14
	NE+PSG	NE+VAFSG	-0.14	0.21	0.97

Fig. 4.50 Mean Serum Globulin in pre-school children during different stages of interventions

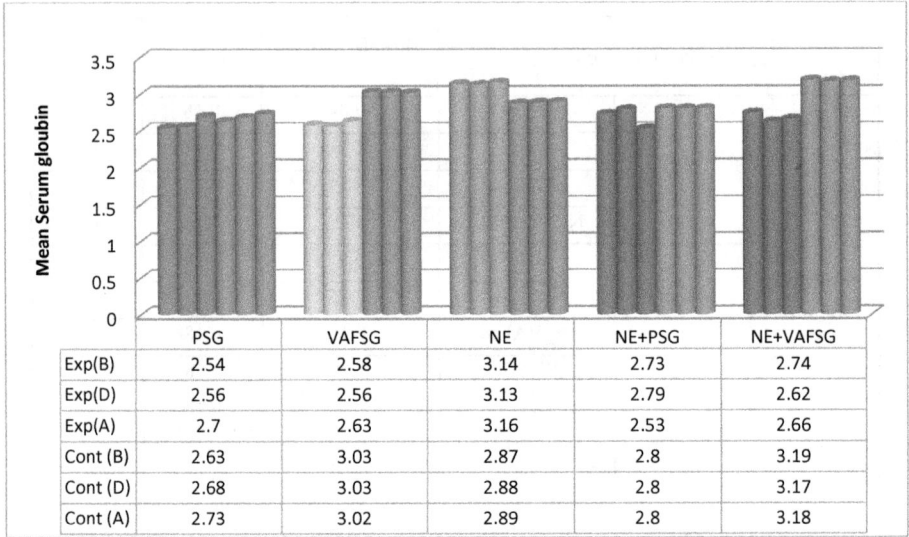

	PSG	VAFSG	NE	NE+PSG	NE+VAFSG
Exp(B)	2.54	2.58	3.14	2.73	2.74
Exp(D)	2.56	2.56	3.13	2.79	2.62
Exp(A)	2.7	2.63	3.16	2.53	2.66
Cont (B)	2.63	3.03	2.87	2.8	3.19
Cont (D)	2.68	3.03	2.88	2.8	3.17
Cont (A)	2.73	3.02	2.89	2.8	3.18

Fig. 4.51 Per cent change in Serum Globulin in pre-school children before, during and after intervention

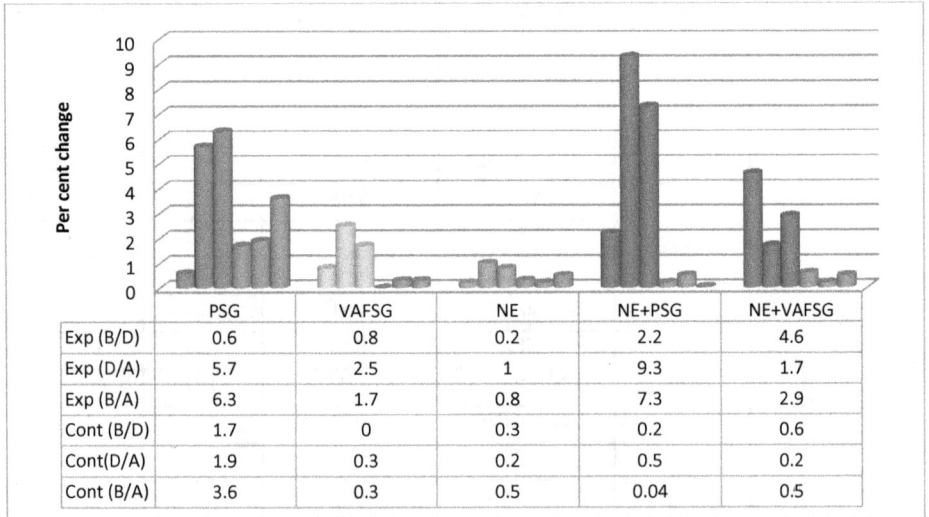

	PSG	VAFSG	NE	NE+PSG	NE+VAFSG
Exp (B/D)	0.6	0.8	0.2	2.2	4.6
Exp (D/A)	5.7	2.5	1	9.3	1.7
Exp (B/A)	6.3	1.7	0.8	7.3	2.9
Cont (B/D)	1.7	0	0.3	0.2	0.6
Cont(D/A)	1.9	0.3	0.2	0.5	0.2
Cont (B/A)	3.6	0.3	0.5	0.04	0.5

Table: 4.27 Efficacy of nutrition interventions on the Haemoglobin of the pre-school children during different stages of interventions

Nutrition Interventions		Actual Increase			Mean change								t value		
		Before (0day)	During (60days)	After (120days)	B/D		D/A		B/A				B/D (0-60 days)	D/A (60-120 days)	B/A (0-120 days)
					Total	%	Total	%	Total	%					
PSG	Control	8.56±1.58	8.60±1.44	8.76±1.41	0.04	0.5	0.16	1.9	0.2	2.3			0.210	1.090	1.360
	Experimental	8.71±1.12	8.86±1.13	9.67±1.06	0.16	1.8	0.81	9.1	0.97	11.1			1.24	4.19**	4.40**
VAFSG	Control	8.14±1.05	8.31±0.97	7.97±1.06	0.17	2.1	0.34	4.1	0.17	2.1			1.14	2.80*	1.19
	Experimental	8.84±1.85	9.35±1.68	10.42±1.52	0.51	5.8	1	11.5	1.59	17.9			4.31**	8.41**	11.21**
N.E	Control	8.66±0.92	8.65±0.74	8.53±0.75	0.01	0.1	0.12	1.3	0.13	1.4			0.1	1.19	1.12
	Experimental	8.66±1.45	8.93±1.28	9.45±1.05	0.27	3.1	0.52	5.8	0.79	9.1			1.64	3.73**	5.16**
N.E+PSG	Control	8.25±0.91	8.22±0.92	8.21±0.87	0.04	0.4	0.01	0.1	0.04	0.5			0.29	0.04	0.28
	Experimental	8.80±1.27	10.33±1.01	11.06±0.94	1.53	17.4	0.73	7.1	2.26	25.7			6.65**	4.42**	7.80**
N.E+ VAFSG	Control	8.36±1.03	8.39±0.89	8.20±1.05	0.03	0.3	0.19	2.3	0.16	2			0.32	1.95	2.03
	Experimental	9.75±1.62	9.87±1.37	11.01±1.09	0.12	1.3	1.14	11.6	1.27	13			0.8	10.28**	7.09**

**significant at p≤0.01, *significant at p≤ 0.05

CONTROL– No Intervention

PSG- Probiotic supplemented group; VAFSG –Value-added food supplemented group; NE –Nutrition education; NE+PSG- Nutrition education+ Probiotic supplemented group; NE +VAFSG – Nutrition education + value -added food supplemented group

B/D – Before / During D/A- During/ After B/A– Before/ After

129

4.5.12 Efficacy of nutrition interventions on Haemoglobin of the pre-school children

PSG: The respective mean haemoglobin values in the probiotic supplemented experimental and control sub-groups were 8.71±1.12g, 8.86±1.13g, 9.67±1.06g and 8.56±1.58g, 8.60±1.44g, 8.76±1.41g at 0 days, 60 days and 120 days of the intervention trial period. In control sub-group, 2.3 per cent change was noticed in respect of haemoglobin parameter, While, a mean per cent change of 9.1per cent and 11.1 per cent, respectively for during (60days) and after (120days) was observed and corresponding t static was found to be significantly ($p \leq 0.01$) increased for both (during and after) in the experimental trial. It indicates that the probiotic supplementation was contributing towards improvement in haemoglobin level after 60 and 120 days of supplementation.

VAFSG: Based on the data collected, the average haemoglobin values of the respondents in the experimental sub-group showed an increased mean for during (60days) and after (120days) the nutrition intervention i.e. from 8.84±1.85g to 9.35±1.68g and 10.42±1.52g. As represented table 4.27, among experimental sub-group subjects increased percentage mean of 17.9 per cent, 11.5 per cent and 5.8 per cent at 120 days (B/A), 60 days (D/A) and0 day (B/D), respectively showed statistically significant ($p \leq 0.01$) improvements. Control sub-group subject's mean haemoglobin values of 8.14±1.05g, 8.31±0.97g, and 7.97±1.06g (table 4.27) depicted significant per cent change of 4.1 during D/A with t static of 2.80 ($p \leq 0.01$). Further analysis confirmed the contribution of value added food supplementation trial as a quiet effective in enhancing mean haemoglobin per cent level during all the three stages in the studied sample. The result indicated that there was comparatively highly significant ($p \leq 0.01$) increment in haemoglobin indicator of the respondents after feeding them with value-added food as compared to routine diet. The findings supported the study and showed that there was 13.2 per cent of increment in the experimental group whereas routine diet found only 2.7 per cent of increment (Anitha, 2021).

NE: The respective mean haemoglobin values of the experimental and control sub-groups were 8.66±1.45g, 8.93±1.28g, 9.45±1.05 and 8.66±0.92g, 8.65±0.74g, 8.53±0.75g at before during and after nutrition education intervention trial period. Control sub-group depicted no significant effect but for experimental group, statistically significant ($p \leq 0.01$) changes of 5.8 per cent and 9.1 per cent was observed respectively after 60 days and 120 days of trial period. Perusal of the data revealed some positive impact of nutrition education trial on haemoglobin level of the children which can be acknowledged.

NE+PSG: The data generated showed improving average haemoglobin values among the experimental sub-group subjects i.e. from 8.80±1.27g to 10.33±1.01g, and 11.06±0.94g towards the completion of the trial period. Whereas, for control group respective average haemoglobin values were 8.25±0.91g, 8.22±0.92g, and 8.21±0.87g depicting negligible mean per cent change. Highly improved change in mean per cent i.e. 25.7 per cent (0-120) days and 17.4 per cent (0-60) days was noticed among children intervened with nutrition education and probiotic supplementation. Highly significant (p≤0.01) haemoglobin increment in all the phases of experimental trial interpreted this intervention to be most effective in the sample of the study area.

NE+VAFSG: The observed haemoglobin mean values of the experimental sub-group during different stages of trial period (9.75±1.62g, 9.87±1.37g, 11.01±1.09g) represented improving behaviour during the experimentation period. In the control sub-group as steady improvement was not noticed (8.36±1.03g, 8.39±0.89g, and 8.20±1.05g), hence no significant change at any stage of the study period was observed. Among experimental sub-group, maximum mean per cent change of 11.6% and 13% in haemoglobin was obtained for two phases i.e. during (60days) and after (120days) the supplementation trial respectively. Highly significant (p≤0.01) increment during and after the supplementation trial in the experimental sub-group indicated relative effectiveness of intervention trial.

Durairaj, (2019) also indicated that haemoglobin and anthropometric parameters of pre-school children increased after supplemented with millet-pulse mixture. It was found that only experimental group has increment when compared with control.

The analysis through application of paired t test revealed that the control sub-group of VAFSG for D/A (60-120days) was significant at 5 per cent; the rest of other respective control samples were not showing any significant impact of nutrition interventions on mean haemoglobin level. Experimental sub-groups of PSG, NE and NE+VAFSG showed significant improvement after 60-120 and after 120 complete days of intervention, whereas experimental sub-group of VAFSG and NE+PSG represented significant improvement at all the three stages of intervention trial i.e. after 60, 60-120 and 120 days. The study has clearly indicated that nutrition interventions of almost all the experimental sub-groups have shown favourable results and can be taken as a good response of nutrition interventions in the study area.

Haemoglobin, one of the most important indicators has been observed to be affected by the nutritional interventions. The table 4.27 suggested that the highest mean percentage change in haemoglobin of the order of 25.7 per cent was identified in the experimental sample of NE+PSG. This indicates that this nutrition intervention has affected most in the experimental sample compared to all other interventions. Apart from this intervention sub-group, some others have also shown good impact i.e. 17.9% by VAFSG, 13% by NE+ VAFSG and 11.1% by PSG. As it evident through highly significant values of t-static ($p \leq 0.01$) that NE+PSG and VAFSG have shown much greater impact as seen during the entire experiment period and could be regarded as real effects of nutrition interventions in the study area.

Table 4.28 Analysis of Variance for Haemoglobin before during and after intervention

	Before						During						After				
	SS	DF	MS	F	P		SS	DF	MS	F	P		SS	DF	MS	F	P
Between Groups	16.268	4	4.067			Between Groups	31.513	4	7.878			Between Groups	44.289	4	11.072		
Within Groups	210.282	95	2.213	1.837	0.128	Within Groups	165.715	95	1.744	4.516	0.002	Within Groups	126.431	95	1.331	8.32	<0.001
Total	226.55	99				Total	197.228	99				Total	170.72	99			

The perusal of the data in Table 4.28 revealed that analysis of variance for haemoglobin showed highly significant (p<0.01) improvement among all the experimental subjects on various nutrition interventions after 2 and 4months of intervention trial. Analysis by Tukey HSD test (Table 4.29) showed that a significant difference was observed in between PSG and NE+PSG, in between VAFSG and NE+VAFSG, in between NE and NE+VAFSG, in between NE+PSG and NE+VAFSG in the mid (0-60 days) of the experimental trial. Significant improvement was noticed at 60-120 days of experimental trial in between PSG and NE+PSG, NE+VAFSG in between VAFSG and PSG, in between NE and NE+PSG, NE+VAFSG respectively. Further after 120 days a highly significant (p< 0.01) increment was noticed for haemoglobin in between PSG and NE+PSG, NE+VAFSG , in between VAFSG and NE, in between NE and NE+PSG, NE+VAFSG.

Table 4.29 Multiple Comparisons for Haemoglobin of pre-school children before, during and after nutrition interventions Tukey HSD

	Dependent Variable		Mean Difference (I-J)	Std. Error	P Value
HB Before	PSG	VAFSG	-0.13	0.47	1
		NE	0.04	0.47	1
		NE+PSG	-0.09	0.47	1
		NE+VAFSG	-1.04	0.47	0.18
	VAFSG	NE	0.18	0.47	1
		NE+PSG	0.04	0.47	1
		NE+VAFSG	-0.91	0.47	0.31
	NE	NE+PSG	-0.13	0.47	1
		NE+VAFSG	-1.09	0.47	0.15
	NE+PSG	NE+VAFSG	-0.95	0.47	0.26
HB During	PSG	VAFSG	-0.48	0.42	0.77
		NE	-0.06	0.42	1
		NE+PSG	-1.46*	0.42	0.01
		NE+VAFSG	-1.01	0.42	0.12
	VAFSG	NE	0.42	0.42	0.85
		NE+PSG	-0.98	0.42	0.14
		NE+VAFSG	-0.52	0.42	0.72
	NE	NE+PSG	-1.40*	0.42	0.01
		NE+VAFSG	-0.94	0.42	0.17
	N E+PSG	NE+VAFSG	0.46	0.42	0.81
HB After	PSG	VAFSG	-0.75	0.36	0.25
		NE	0.23	0.36	0.97
		NE+PSG	-1.38*	0.36	0
		NE+VAFSG	-1.34*	0.36	0
	VAFSG	NE	0.97	0.36	0.07
		NE+PSG	-0.64	0.36	0.41
		NE+VAFSG	-0.59	0.36	0.49
	NE	NE+PSG	-1.61*	0.36	0
		NE+VAFSG	-1.56*	0.36	0
	NE+ PSG	NE+VAFSG	0.04	0.36	1

Fig. 4.52 Mean Haemoglobin of pre-school children during different stages of nutrition interventions

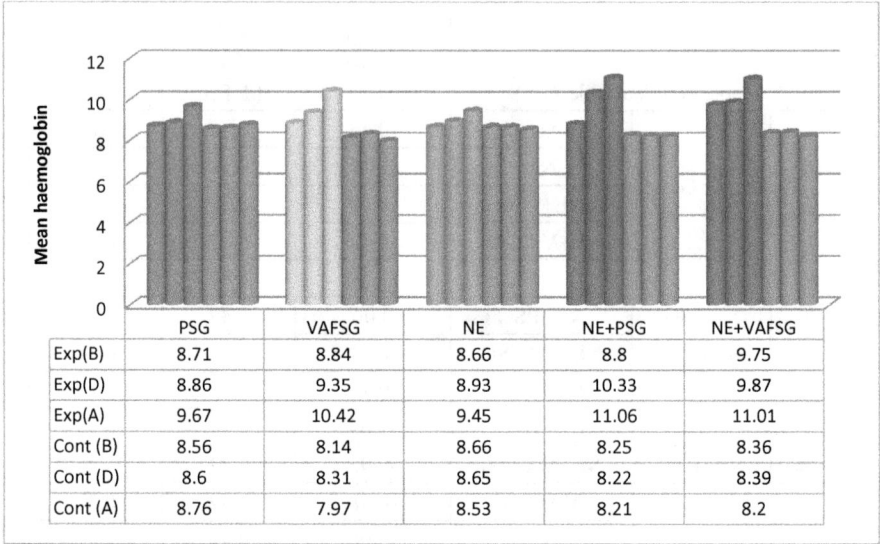

	PSG	VAFSG	NE	NE+PSG	NE+VAFSG
Exp(B)	8.71	8.84	8.66	8.8	9.75
Exp(D)	8.86	9.35	8.93	10.33	9.87
Exp(A)	9.67	10.42	9.45	11.06	11.01
Cont (B)	8.56	8.14	8.66	8.25	8.36
Cont (D)	8.6	8.31	8.65	8.22	8.39
Cont (A)	8.76	7.97	8.53	8.21	8.2

Fig. 4.53 Per cent change Haemoglobin in pre-school children before, during and after intervention

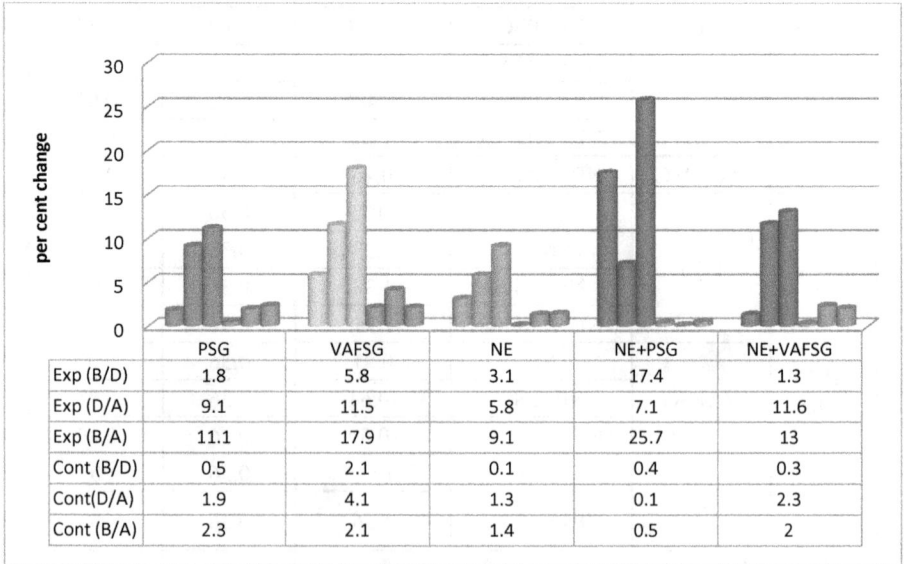

	PSG	VAFSG	NE	NE+PSG	NE+VAFSG
Exp (B/D)	1.8	5.8	3.1	17.4	1.3
Exp (D/A)	9.1	11.5	5.8	7.1	11.6
Exp (B/A)	11.1	17.9	9.1	25.7	13
Cont (B/D)	0.5	2.1	0.1	0.4	0.3
Cont(D/A)	1.9	4.1	1.3	0.1	2.3
Cont (B/A)	2.3	2.1	1.4	0.5	2

4.6 Assessment of Knowledge, Attitude, and Practice Scores of nutrition education among mothers

During the experimentation it was through to study the behaviour indicators of mothers of the children under study who were imparted nutrition education for the future all round development in the children. Three groups namely NE, NE+PSG, and NE+VAFSG were subjected to study the knowledge, attitude and practice of the concerned mothers. Personal interview method was adopted to record the data as per group on NE, NE+PSG and NE+VAFSG in respect of mothers under study. The scoring was carried out before and after the experiment further analysed statistically to draw logical inferences.

Nutrition Education: The mean knowledge, attitude and practice scores of the mothers before imparting nutrition education to the experimental group were 1.60±1.23, 1.85±1.38 and 1.60±1.31 respectively. At the end of the experiment an increment in mean per cent change was 340.62, 316.21 and 406.25 per cent. Statistically t value showed highly significant (p≤0.01) difference between before and after clearly indicating the effect of NE on the gain in knowledge, attitude and practice in the experimental group. KAP scores in respect of NE for control group were estimated as 0.55±0.68, 10.70±0.86 and 10.90±0.64 respectively with negative per cent change of -36.36, -1.86 and -2.09 after study period. Since the test has not shown gain in knowledge in the control subjects (mothers of the subjects). A study was carried out by Yetnayet *et.al* (2017) in district Hawassa Zuria in Ethiopia. The calculated results of the study revealed significant (p≤0.01) improvement in mean KAP scores of the experiment trial group in comparison with control group after imparting nutrition education.

NE+PSG: Mean KAP scores of NE+PSG experimental group before and after nutrition education were 1.15±0.93, 11.05±0.88, 11.95±1.53 and 7.45±1.23, 17.40±1.39, 18.00±1.33, respectively. Mean per cent change was maximum for knowledge scores (547.8%) followed by 57.46 and 50.6 per cent for attitude and practice scores, respectively. Further analysis through t values showed highly significant (p≤0.01) change in before (0day) and after (120days) the intervention trial. Experimental group of NE+PSG showed sufficient gain in knowledge, attitude and practice. While in control group of NE+PSG the mean knowledge score had shown a per cent gain of 50 per cent but statistically non-significant. No change was noticed in the mean scores of practice and attitude scores among control group mothers.

135

Table 4.30 Mean in knowledge, attitude and practice scores before and after imparting nutrition education

Experimental Groups		Knowledge	Attitude	Practice
Nutrition Education	**Control**			
	Before	0.55±0.68	10.70±0.86	10.90±0.64
	After	0.35±0.48	10.50±0.60	10.65±0.58
	Mean Change	-0.2 (-36.36)	-0.2 (-1.86)	-0.25 (-2.09)
	t value	1.07	0.89	1.31
	Experimental			
	Before	1.60±1.23	11.85±1.38	11.60±1.31
	After	7.05±1.14	17.70±1.17	18.10±1.2
	Mean Change	5.45 (340.62)	5.85 (48.94)	6.5 (56.0)
	t value	15.84**	12.25**	16.78**
NE+PSG	**Control**			
	Before	0.2±0.41	10.50±0.76	11.10±1.02
	After	0.30±0.57	10.60±0.99	11.10±0.85
	Mean Change	0.1 (50)	0.1 (0.95)	0 (0)
	t value	0.8	0.62	0
	Experimental			
	Before	1.15±0.93	11.05±0.88	11.95±1.53
	After	7.45±1.23	17.40±1.39	18.00±1.33
	Mean Change	6.3 (547.8)	6.35 (57.46)	6.05 (50.6)
	t value	22.34**	18.97**	13.80**
NE+VAFSG	**Control**			
	Before	0.25±0.44	10.90±0.55	11.10±0.85
	After	0.05±0.22	10.90±0.71	11.05±0.88
	Mean Change	0.2 (-5)	0 (0)	0.05 (0.45)
	t value	1.71	0	0.29
	Experimental			
	Before	1.45±0.99	11.40±0.99	11.55±1.09
	After	6.95±1.57	18.40±1.04	17.85±1.22
	Mean Change	5.5 (379.3)	7(61.4)	6.3 (54.5)
	t value	12.21**	20.11**	17.33**

NE+VAFSG: Before commencing the experimental trial, mean KAP scores were 1.45±0.99, 11.40±0.99 and 11.55±1.09, respectively. At the end (120 days) of experimental trial their mean scores were 6.95±1.57, 18.40±1.04 and 17.85±1.22 respectively. The results of experimental group revealed that there was gain of 379.3 per cent in knowledge scores, 61.4 per cent change for attitude scores and 54.5 per cent of increment in attitude. The t values for the entire three attribute found to be highly significant (p≤0.01). In respect of control group, change of zero-order clearly explaining the fact that the knowledge, attitude and practices has not at all improved during the experimental period of 120 days. The study indicating that from beginning to the end of experiment the practices being followed in control group was unchanged.

Likewise, Mochoni, (2020) reported that there was a significant change in mean scores (knowledge) of experiment trial group and also concluded that maximum mother had gain good knowledge on complementary feeding after given them nutrition education as compared to control group. Similar study carried out by Teshome, (2020) revealed an increase in weight of children after imparting nutrition education on complementary feeding. A significant improvement (p≤0.001) in the KAP scores and the occurrence of stunting, wasting and underweight was declined in the intervention trial group in contrast to control group. Aguayo, (2017) also suggested a need to elevate the knowledge of mothers so that they feed healthy diet to the children for healthy future.

Kaur *et.al*, (2007) reported in their study that nutrition education was effectual in gaining nutritional knowledge as well as the daily intake of nutrients. The similar finding of Yetnayet *et al.,* (2017) indicated a significant increment (p≤0.001) in the mean KAP scores of experimental group.

The study conducted by Naghashpour *et.al*, (2014) reported that there was an increment in KAP scores of the respondents after imparting nutrition education. Another experimental study by Anand and Anuradha (2018) findings revealed that there was significant improvement (p≤0.001) in the KAP scores when compared to control group. The results showed gain in knowledge, practice and attitude scores (10.24, 10.28 and 9.12).

Fig.4.54 Distribution of mean knowledge scores of the mothers

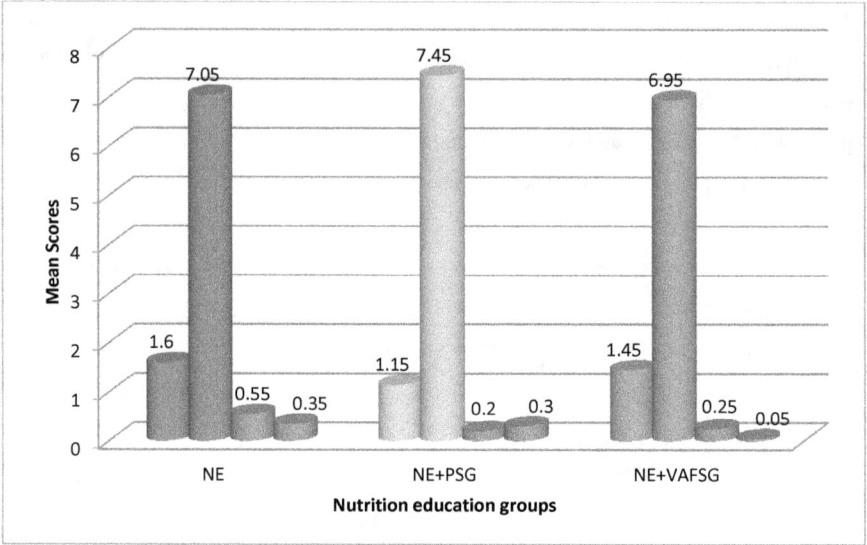

Fig.4.55 Distribution of mean attitude scores of the mothers

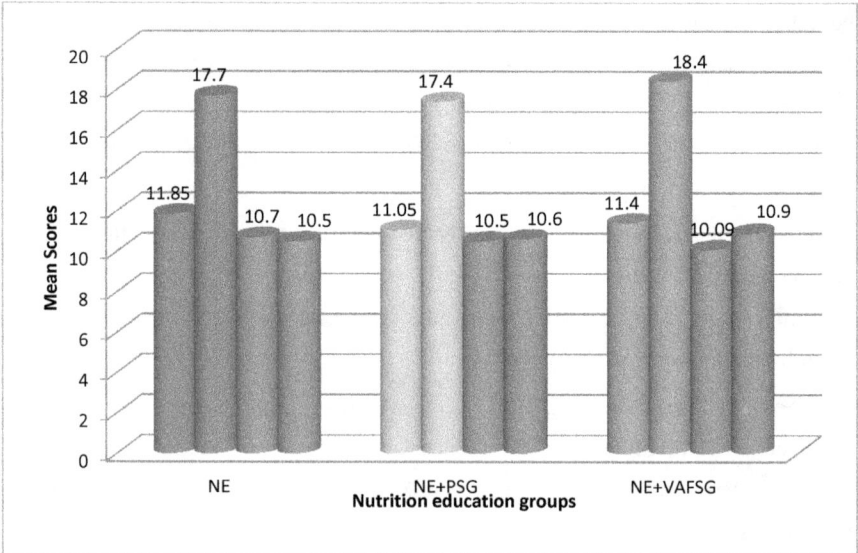

Fig.4.56 Distribution of mean practice scores of the mothers

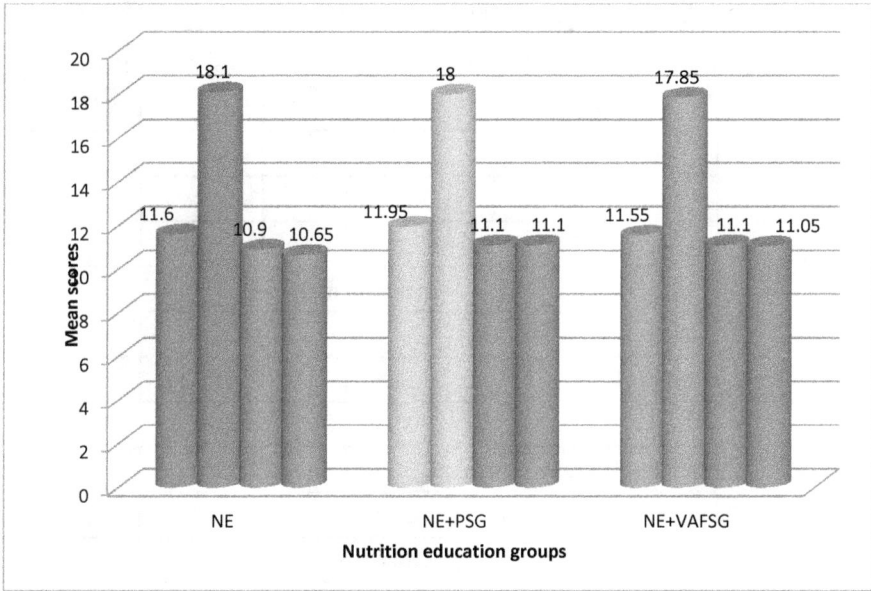

Fig.4.56 Distribution of mean practice scores of the mothers

Fig.4.57 Distribution of Mean per cent change in KAP scores of the mothers

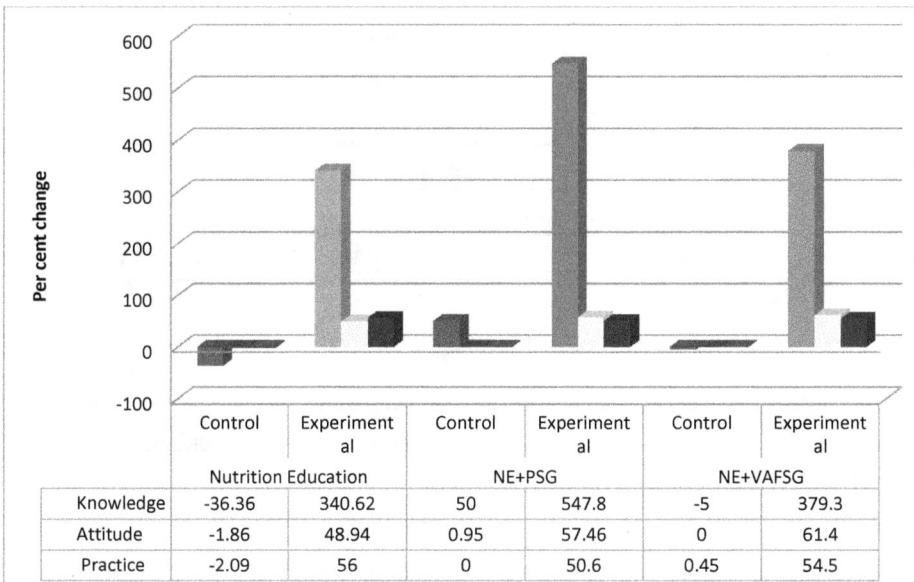

Fig.4.57 Distribution of Mean per cent change in KAP scores of the mothers

	Control	Experimental	Control	Experimental	Control	Experimental
	Nutrition Education		NE+PSG		NE+VAFSG	
Knowledge	-36.36	340.62	50	547.8	-5	379.3
Attitude	-1.86	48.94	0.95	57.46	0	61.4
Practice	-2.09	56	0	50.6	0.45	54.5

4.31 Nutrition KAP (knowledge, attitude and practice) scores of the mothers before and after imparting nutrition education

Nutrition interventions		Very poor (0.5)	Poor (6-10)	Average (11-15)	Good (16-20)	Very Good (21-25)	Excellent (26-30)
N.E	Control						
	Before	20 (100)	.....	.....	.....	.....	.....
	After	20 (100)	.....	.....	.....	.....	.....
	Experimental						
	Before	13 (65)	7 (35)	.....	.....	.....	.....
	After	.....	.....	.....	3 (15)	15 (75)	2 (10)
N.E+PSG	Control						
	Before	19 (95)	1 (5)	.....	.....	.....	.....
	After	19 (95)	1 (5)	.....	.....	.....	.....
	Experimental						
	Before	15(75)	5 (25)	.....	.....	.....	.....
	After	.....	.....	.....	6 (30)	10 (50)	4 (20)
N.E+VAFSG	Control						
	Before	20 (100)	.....	.....	.....	.....	.....
	After	20 (100)	.....	.....	.....	.....	.....
	Experimental						
	Before	13 (65)	7 (35)	.....	.....	.....	.....
	After	.....	.....	.....	3 (15)	13 (65)	4 (20)

Figures in parenthesis are in percentage

4.6.1 Nutrition KAP (knowledge, attitude and practice) scores of the mothers

100 per cent of the mothers of NE control group were scored very poor grades before and after experimental trial, (Table 4.31). Before imparting nutrition education in the experimental group, majority (65%) of the children mothers scored very poor marks and almost $1/3^{rd}$ of the subjects scored marks in between 6-10(poor). After 120 days of imparting nutrition education to the mothers the categories of scores was improved. Out of total, 10 per cent fell in the excellent scores (26-30) category whereas $3/4^{th}$ of

the mothers scored very good marks (21-25) and 30 per cent scored good marks (16-20). The results of experimental trial showed that there was an effect of nutrition education interventions on the mothers of the respondents. N.E+PSG control group reported that 95 per cent of the mothers got very poor (0-5) scores and 1 per cent mothers scored poor (6-10) marks and the percentage remained same after 120 days trial period. Among the NE+PSG group it was found experimental found that 3/4th of the mothers scored very poor scores and 1/4th got poor marks. However after four months of nutrition intervention trial there was an increment of scores hence shifted to better category. Half (50%) of the mothers scored very good (21-25) marks, 1/5th of the mothers scored excellent (26-30) marks and 30 per cent scored good (16-20) marks. All the mothers of control group of NE+VAFSG scored very poor (0-5) marks before and after four months of experimental trial. The scores of experimental group was almost similar to NE+PSG experimental group, 65 and 35 per cent of the mothers were in very poor and poor marks category, respectively. The scores of all the mothers improved and moved in superior category of scores i.e.20 per cent of the mother scored excellent marks followed by very good (65%) and good marks (15%), after intervention period.

The findings of Mochoni, (2020) reported that the audio-visual aids play a major part in imparting knowledge and in changing the behaviour of individual on value-added feeding. Oli *et.al*,(2018) assessed the knowledge of mothers based on the different categories (poor, fair and good) of scores and result of the study concluded that all the mothers of the respondents were in fair and poor category scores. A study was conducted on 160 mother's to evaluate Knowledge, attitude and practice scores before and after experiment. The result revealed that the KAP scores of the mothers increased significantly ($p \leq 0.05$) as compared to control group. Significant improvement in mean change was also observed in weight-for-age, and weight-for-height of children. There also improvement in nutrition status of children who were intervened with pulse-based nutrition education (Mulualem, 2016). A study was carried out to assess the knowledge of the mothers of children less than 5 years by Shettigar, (2013) the data revealed that 54 per cent had poor knowledge whereas 38 per cent had average knowledge and only 8 per cent had good knowledge

Fig.4.58 Nutrition KAP scores obtained by the mothers of pre-school children before and after nutrition education

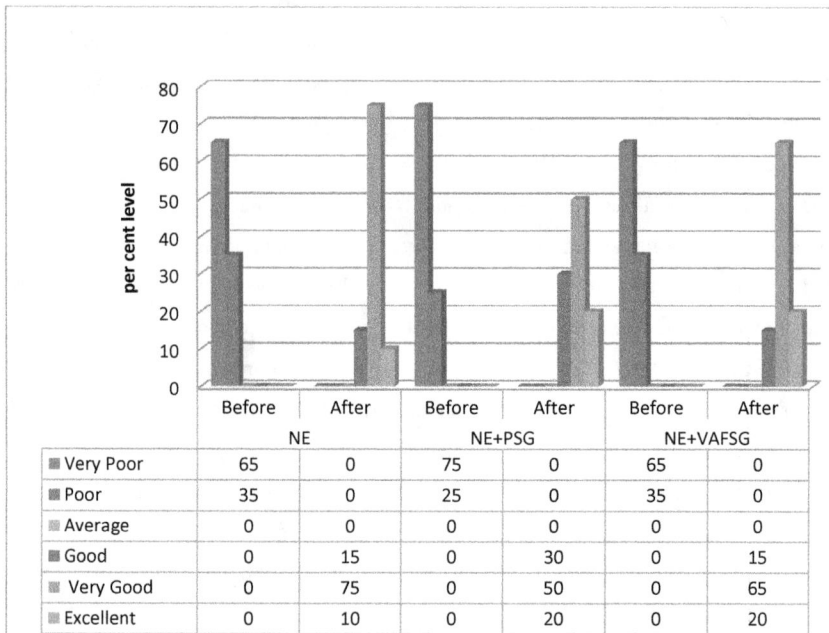

	Before	After	Before	After	Before	After
	NE		NE+PSG		NE+VAFSG	
▦ Very Poor	65	0	75	0	65	0
▦ Poor	35	0	25	0	35	0
▦ Average	0	0	0	0	0	0
▦ Good	0	15	0	30	0	15
▦ Very Good	0	75	0	50	0	65
▦ Excellent	0	10	0	20	0	20

4.7 Prevalence of undernutrition among pre-school children

Malnutrition is a phenomenon that affects the overall development of a child. In the present investigation, pre-school children were classified according to age as 3, 4, 5, and 6 years. To assess the malnutrition effects in these categories of sample children, the factors like age, height, and weight, It is assuming that these variables under study follow in the normal distribution and the classification according to low, moderate, and severe malnutrition effect can be measured using normalized Z- scores and can be safely interpreted for their malnourishment.

In the present research problem, there are three variables under study, namely viz;

1. Weight for age (underweight)
2. Height for age (stunted)
3. Weight-for-height (wasted)

The WHO criterion of classification based on Z score was used to identify undernutrition among the sample children of 200 hundred. The individual children

142

were segregated based on the Z score so calculated and the criterion adopted was

1. Z= -2 to +2 SD (Normal)
2. Z= < -2 SD (Moderately malnourished)
3. Z = < -3SD (Severely malnourished)

Weight for age: Age-wise prevalence data revealed that in the 3 years age group one half (51.4%) of experimental and most of (46.66%) of the control subjects were severely underweight, while 40 and 41.66 per cent were moderately underweight in the experimental and control group, respectively. Only 8.57 per cent and 16.66 per cent subjects in the corresponding groups belonged to normal category. For 4 years age group maximum (89.74%) of the pre-school children in the experimental group and all (100%) of the respondents in the control group were reported severely underweight. All the respondents (100%) of experimental and control group of 5 and 6 years of age group were assessed as severely underweight. Likewise a study was conducted to assess the prevalence of undernutrition among children (less than 5 years) in the two different region of Maharashtra and the study revealed that 45.9, 17.1 and 35.4 per cent of children were stunted, wasting and underweight respectively (Murarkar,2020).

Height for age: As per height for age data, the findings revealed that most of the pre-school children of experimental group 3 years age-group were severely stunted (37.14%) followed by normal (34.28%) and moderately stunted (28.57%). Most of control group children were in normal category (54.16%) followed by moderate (41.66%) and only 4.16 were severely undernourished.

In the experimental group among 4 years of age-group, maximum (79.48%) respondents were severely stunted while equal percentage (10.25% each) of the pre-schoolers fell in moderate and normal category, whereas in the control group all the subjects were severely stunted. All most all the pre-schoolers of 5 and 6 years of the age group were severely stunted and only 10 per cent of the experimental subjects in 6 years age-group were moderately stunted.

Weight-for-height: The data for weight-for-height revealed that 22.85 per cent and 37.5 per cent of the preschool children of 3 years age group in the experimental and control were severely wasted, and at the same time 34.28 per cent in experimental and 33.33 per cent in control group found to be moderately wasted respectively. For 4 years age group 17.94 and 41.17 per cent of the subjects were severely wasted in experimental and control group, respectively. While 35.89 per cent of subjects in the experimental group were moderately wasted as depicted in the table 4.32. In the control group same (29.4%) per cent of the respondents were falling in moderate and normal category each. For 5 years age-group maximum (56.25% and 46.42%) of the subjects were severely and moderately wasted in experimental and control group, respectively. 2/5th of the experimental subjects were severely and moderately wasted and only 20 per cent were in normal category. However equal (25.80%) percentage of the control subjects falling in severe and normal category, whereas a maximum (48.38%) per cent of control subjects were moderately wasted. Huey *et.al*,(2019) conducted study on young children of slum areas to record prevalence of undernutrition. The result revealed that 31.2 per cent children were stunted whereas 25.1 per cent were underweight and 9 per cent were wasted

Table 4.32 Prevalence of undernutrition among the pre-school children before imparting nutrition intervention

Age	Groups	Weight-for-age (Underweight)			Height-for-age (Stunting)			Weight-for-height (wasting)		
		-2.0 to 2.0 SD	<-2.0 SD	<-3.0 SD	-2.0 to 2.0 SD	<-2.0 SD	<-3.0 SD	-2.0 to 2.0 SD	<-2.0 SD	<-3.0 SD
3 years	Experimental	8.57	40	51.42	34.28	28.57	37.14	42.85	34.28	22.85
	Control	16.66	41.66	41.66	54.16	41.66	4.16	29.16	33.33	37.5
4 years	Experimental	2.56	7.69	89.74	10.25	10.25	79.48	46.15	35.89	17.94
	Control	-	-	100	-	-	100	29.41	29.41	41.17
5 years	Experimental	-	-	100	-	6.25	93.75	37.5	56.25	6.25
	Control	-	-	100	-	3.57	96.42	14.28	39.28	46.42
6 years	Experimental	-	-	100	-	10	90	20	40	40
	Control	-	-	100	-	-	100	25.80	48.38	25.80

Figures in parenthesis are in percentage

Table 4.33 Prevalence of WAZ, HAZ and WHZ in pre-school children before and after imparting nutrition interventions

Age	Groups		Weight-for-age(Underweight)			Height-for-age(Stunting)			Weight-for-height(Wasting)		
			-2.0 to 2.0 SD	<-2.0 SD	<-3.0 SD	-2.0 to 2.0 SD	<-2.0 SD	<-3.0 SD	-2.0 to 2.0 SD	<-2.0 SD	<-3.0 SD
3 years	Experimental	Before	8.57	40	51.42	34.28	28.57	37.14	42.85	34.28	22.85
		After	54.28	45.71	-	40	48.57	11.4	91.42	5.71	2.85
	Control	Before	16.66	41.66	41.66	54.16	41.66	4.16	29.16	33.33	37.5
		After	20.83	45.83	33.33	58.33	41.66	-	37.5	37.5	25
4 years	Experimental	Before	2.56	7.69	89.74	10.25	10.25	79.48	46.15	35.89	17.94
		After	15.38	43.58	41.02	10.25	7.69	82.05	84.31	7.69	7.69
	Control	Before	-	-	100	-	-	100	29.41	29.41	41.17
		After	-	-	100	-	-	100	35.29	41.17	23.52
5 years	Experimental	Before	-	-	100	-	6.25	93.75	37.5	56.25	6.25
		After	-	37.5	62.5	-	12.5	87.5	87.5	12.5	-
	Control	Before	-	-	100	-	3.57	96.42	14.28	39.28	46.42
		After	-	3.57	96.42	-	3.57	96.42	3.57	39.28	57.14
6 years	Experimental	Before	-	-	100	-	10	90	20	40	40
		After	10	30	60	-	10	90	80	10	10
	Control	Before	-	-	100	-	-	100	25.80	48.38	25.80
		After	-	-	100	-	-	100	29.0	41.93	29.0

Figures in *parenthesis are in percentage

4.7.1 Prevalence of WAZ, HAZ and WHZ in pre-school children before and after imparting nutrition intervention

Weight-for-age: Supplementation had good impact as indicated in the table (4.33). In 3 years age group before supplementation only 8.57 per cent were under normal category, whereas 40 and 51.42 per cent children were moderate and severely underweight, respectively. After supplementation none of the pre-school children was severely underweight as compared to more than one half (51.42%) before supplementation. Majority (54.28%) of the 3 years pre-school children improved and were categorised under normal category of weight-for-age which was just 8.57 per cent before nutrition intervention trials. In the beginning of the study only 40 per cent preschool children were categorised as moderate underweight which increased to 45.71 per cent after nutrition intervention and this improvement can be justified as shifting from severe underweight category to moderate category. Corresponding control pre-schoolers also showed improvement but that was of very less as compared to experimental group represented in table 4.33 in severe category. Among 4 years experimental pre-schoolers, improvement in the nutritional status was also noticed. Before imparting nutrition interventions, most of the preschool children (89.74%) were severely underweight which reduced to 41.02 per cent after imparting nutrition interventions. Under normal category of weight-for-age of preschool children per cent improvement was noticed from 2.56 to 15.38. Per cent improvement was also observed in moderate category from 7.69 to 43.58 which however can be justified as shifting from severe underweight category towards moderate underweight category. Nil improvement was observed among control subjects of 4 years age-group. All the preschoolers less than 5 years experimental groups were severely underweight before imparting nutrition interventions. Nutrition interventions showed good impact on improving the nutritional status as more than $1/3^{rd}$ preschool children improved from severe underweight category to moderate category. Among respective preschoolers of control group only 3.57 per cent improved from severe to moderate underweight category. Efficacy of imparting nutrition interventions was also observed among the 6 years experimental subjects. After 120 days of nutrition intervention percentage of subjects belonged to severe underweight category reduced from 100 to 60 while 30 and 10 per cent preschoolers improved to moderate underweight category and normal category respectively which was nil before interventions. On the contrary no changes

146

were observed among corresponding control subjects.

Likewise a study was conducted on 500 children (less than 6 years) by Tarun *et.al.* (2016) the study revealed that 43 per cent of the subjects were underweight.

Fig. 4.59 Prevalence of underweight among pre-school children

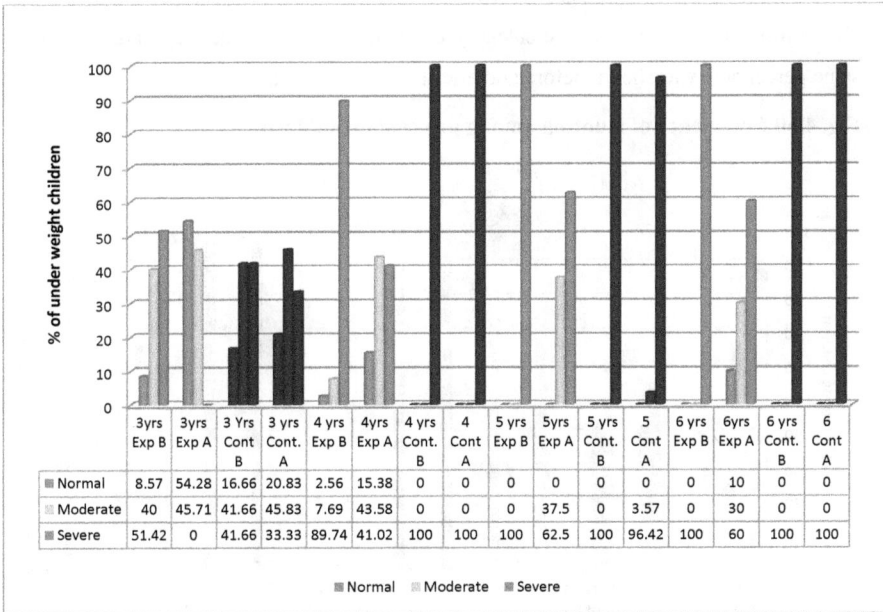

	3yrs Exp B	3yrs Exp A	3 Yrs Cont B	3 yrs Cont. A	4 yrs Exp B	4yrs Exp A	4 yrs Cont. B	4 Cont A	5 yrs Exp B	5yrs Exp A	5 yrs Cont. B	5 Cont A	6 yrs Exp B	6yrs Exp A	6 yrs Cont. B	6 Cont A
▪ Normal	8.57	54.28	16.66	20.83	2.56	15.38	0	0	0	0	0	0	0	10	0	0
▪ Moderate	40	45.71	41.66	45.83	7.69	43.58	0	0	0	37.5	0	3.57	0	30	0	0
▪ Severe	51.42	0	41.66	33.33	89.74	41.02	100	100	100	62.5	100	96.42	100	60	100	100

▪ Normal   ▪ Moderate   ▪ Severe

Height-for-age: As per data collected for height-for-age shown some impact of nutrition intervention on the 3 years of age group pre-school children of experimental group as there were 37.14 per cent of the children were severely malnourished before intervened with supplemented value-added food preparations. However it was declined by 25.74 per cent after the 120 days of experiment. Before intervention only 28.57 per cent and 34.28 per cent subjects were in moderate and normal category. There were an increased percentage of 20 and 5.72 per cent in moderate and normal category which shown different nutrition intervention had some impact on 3 years of children in experimental group. For 4 years age group only 2.21 and 2.56 per cent change was observed for severe and moderate category after the intervention trial. However percentage of normal category was remained same. Among 5 years age-group before supplementation maximum (93.75%) respondents were belonged to severe category and only 6.25 per cent was in normal category. After accomplished the experiment trial 12.5 per cent of the subjects moved from severe category to moderate category of malnourishment. The respondents of 6 years of age group were remained same before and after the trial the reason may be that height growing slower down during that particular age. In case of control group it was observed that almost all the respondents fell in severe category of malnourishment except 3 years and the same percentage was shown before and after the experimentation.

Fig. 4.60 Prevalence of stunting among pre-school children

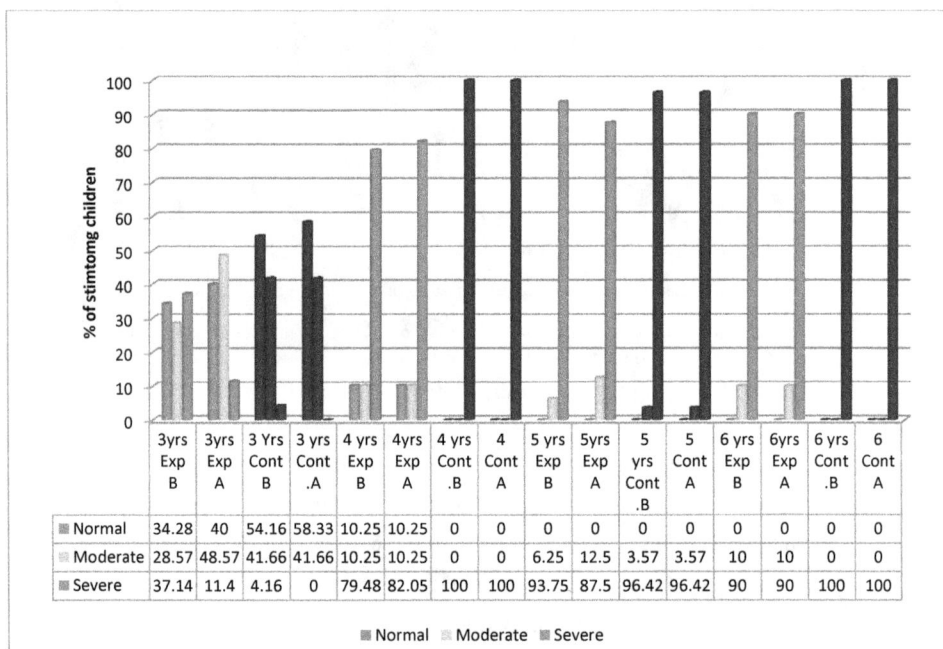

	3yrs Exp B	3yrs Exp A	3 Yrs Cont B	3 yrs Cont .A	4 yrs Exp B	4yrs Exp A	4 yrs Cont .B	4 Cont A	5 yrs Exp B	5yrs Exp A	5 yrs Cont .B	5 Cont A	6 yrs Exp B	6yrs Exp A	6 yrs Cont .B	6 Cont A
Normal	34.28	40	54.16	58.33	10.25	10.25	0	0	0	0	0	0	0	0	0	0
Moderate	28.57	48.57	41.66	41.66	10.25	10.25	0	0	6.25	12.5	3.57	3.57	10	10	0	0
Severe	37.14	11.4	4.16	0	79.48	82.05	100	100	93.75	87.5	96.42	96.42	90	90	100	100

Normal Moderate Severe

Weight-for-height: The distribution of sample units according to age in the experimental group shown that 22.85 per cent of the respondents of 3 years age group were severely malnourished which were left only 2.85 per cent after the experimental trial. 34.28 and 42.85 per cent pre-school children were in moderate malnourished and normal category. Most of (91.42%) the pre-school children moved to normal category after 120 day of experimental trial. Similar trend was observed in experimental group of 4 years. Maximum (84.31%) of the subjects were in normal category after the experimental trial which was 46.15 per cent before the experimental trial. The 35.89 and 17.94 per cent of the subjects were in moderate and severely malnourished category before the experiment started but the percentage of moderate and severe category were decline by 28.2 and 10.25 per cent after intervened with various nutrition interventions. The Weight-for-height of pre-school children of 5 years age group in the experimental group showed that out of total 37.5 per cent were belonged to normal category, more than half (56.25) per cent were moderately malnourished and only 6.25 per cent be in severely malnourished category but after the experimental trial majority (87.5%) of the pre-school children shifted to normal category which showed a good impact of nutrition interventions. Similar trend was noticed in the 6 years of age group where only 20, 40 and 40 per cent of the respondents belonged to normal, moderate and severe category of malnourishment respectively. However out of total maximum (80%) of the respondents fell in normal category. In case of control group there was slight change in percentage except 5 years of age group where the moderate category was remained same before and after experiment however the percentage of the respondents increased in the severe malnourished category after the experimental trial.

A study conducted on preschool children revealed that the prevalence of malnourished children reduced after supplemented them with healthy food preparations. The observed data showed the normal weight-for-age percentage rose from 16.67 per cent to 56.67 per cent. Whereas the percentage of mild malnourished category declined from 83.33 per cent to 43.33 per cent (Dhanesh 2019). The study conducted among 2-5 years children to assess the prevalence of undernutrition the result revealed that 6.3 per cent of the children were underweight (Kumbhar,2018). The findings of the study revealed that overall 46.2 per cent subjects were malnourished. The observed percentage revealed that for weight-for-age 14.5 per cent were underweight and only 4.2 per cent were severely underweight. The prevalence for height-for-age has shown 11.1 per cent were stunted and 4.3 per cent were severely stunted respectively, whereas for BMI-for-age 31.6 and 23.1 per cent subjects were wasted and severely wasted respectively (Tinuola and Olakayode,

2020).The study revealed that the prevalence of child malnutrition in Angola was very high the percentage of underweight children were maximum (95%) where as 32 per cent of the subjects were stunted (Humbwavali, 2019).

Fig. 4.61 Prevalence of wasting among pre-school children

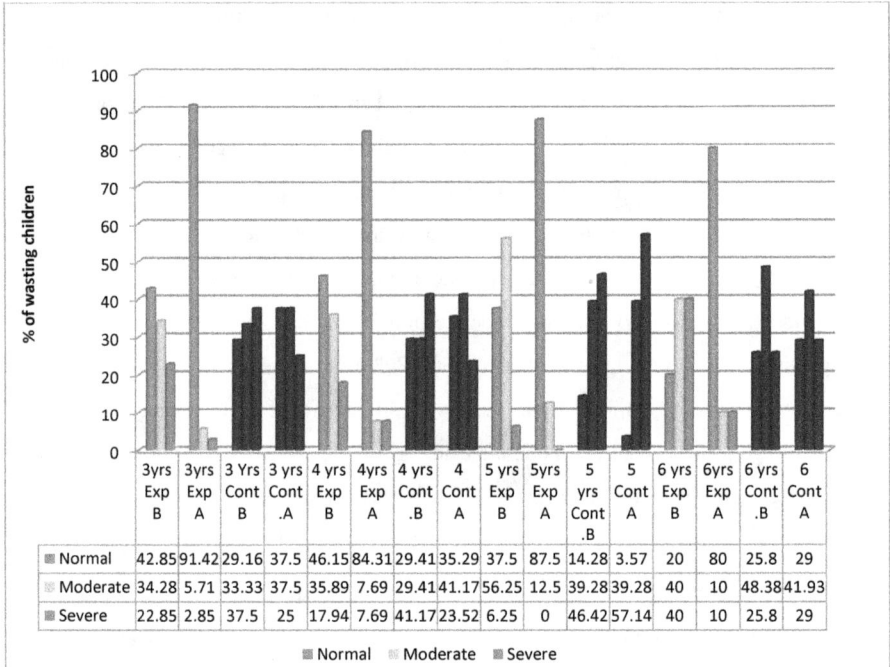

	3yrs Exp B	3yrs Exp A	3 Yrs Cont B	3 yrs Cont .A	4 yrs Exp B	4yrs Exp A	4 yrs Cont .B	4 Cont A	5 yrs Exp B	5yrs Exp A	5 yrs Cont .B	5 Cont A	6 yrs Exp B	6yrs Exp A	6 yrs Cont .B	6 Cont A
Normal	42.85	91.42	29.16	37.5	46.15	84.31	29.41	35.29	37.5	87.5	14.28	3.57	20	80	25.8	29
Moderate	34.28	5.71	33.33	37.5	35.89	7.69	29.41	41.17	56.25	12.5	39.28	39.28	40	10	48.38	41.93
Severe	22.85	2.85	37.5	25	17.94	7.69	41.17	23.52	6.25	0	46.42	57.14	40	10	25.8	29

■ Normal ■ Moderate ■ Severe

Table 4.34 Overall Prevalence of undernutrition in the pre-school children before and after imparting nutrition intervention

Groups		Z -2 to+2 SD (Normal)			Z <-2 SD (Moderate undernourished)			Z <-3 SD (Severely undernourished)		
		Weight-for-age	Height-for-age	Weight-for-height	Weight-for-age	Height-for-age	Weight-for-height	Weight-for-age	Height-for-age	Weight-for-height
Experimental	Before	4	16	41	17	16	39	79	68	20
	After	26	18	87	42	23	8	32	59	5
Control	Before	4	13	24	10	11	39	86	76	37
	After	5	14	25	12	11	40	83	75	35

Figures in parenthesis are in percentage

4.7.2 Overall prevalence of undernutrition in the pre-school children

Weight-for-age: As per data collected overall prevalence of undernutrition after imparting different nutrition interventions the study indicated sharp decrease (47%) in the cases of severe malnourishment after imparting nutrition interventions, which got shifted to moderate (25%) and normal (22%) categories. While in control group there was not much change of percentage before and after intervention trial as presented in table (4.34). Silva *et.al.* (2015) studied prevalence of wasting, stunted and underweight children. The study concluded that 13.8 per cent, 31.2 per cent and 21.4 per cent children were wasted, stunted and underweight, respectively

4.62: Overall Prevalence of underweight among pre-school children.

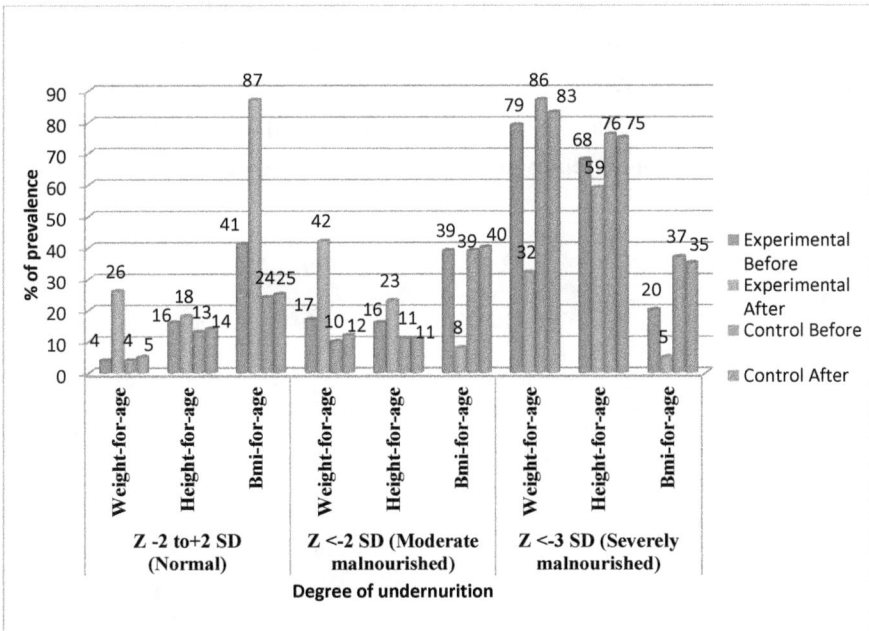

Height-for-age: The percentage for height-for-age revealed that 16, 16 and 68 per cent of the experimental subjects were in the category of normal, moderate and severe malnourished before (0day) imparting nutrition interventions, whereas after (120 days) completion of experimental trial 18, 23 and 59 per cent subjects were in the category of normal, moderate and severe malnourished. In case of control group almost negligible change was found among all the categories of undernutrition in normal and moderate category. Vikas *et.al.* (2015) concluded that prevalence of stunted children was 21.4 per cent in his study.

Weight-for-height: As per weight-for-height revealed that in the experimental group, 46 per cent moved to the normal category of weight-for-height (wasting), out of which 31 per cent were from moderate category and the rest were from severe malnourished category. Only 8 and 5 per cent of the respondents were in moderate and severe category after 120 days of experimental trial. In the control group not much change was noticed before and after the experimental trial period which further showed that nutrition intervention has good impact on weight-for height. Mahalakshmi and Abirami (2019) also reported that gender and the age of the individual has a sturdy impact on BMI. It also concluded that good food and dietary habits required to be modified accordingly. The findings are in accord with the results of Msuda *et.al* (2014) who carried out a study on pre-school malnourished children and intervened them with spirulina rich food preparations and the results showed a significant increment in mid-upper arm circumference, height-for-age and weight-for-age.

SUMMARY

Under-nutrition is the root cause of 45 percent of all infant deaths worldwide. Nearly 4 in 10 children in Sub-Saharan Africa and Asia are stunted–a debilitating illness that restricts the growth of their brains and bodies and also has an impact on almost every aspect of their well-being. Keeping this in view the present research project with following objectives was proposed:

1. To assess nutritional status of undernourished children.
2. To develop enriched food preparations and nutrition education material for nutrition intervention.
3. To intervene undernourished children with nutrition interventions.
4. To study the efficacy of nutrition interventions on nutritional status of undernourished children.

Two hundred undernourished pre-school children randomly selected from Karnal district were stratified into five strata. These strata of forty units, each with twenty control and twenty experimental, constituted the basis of the study. Experimental trials sub-groups were named as per their nutrition intervention viz. Probiotic supplemented group (PSG), Value-added food supplemented group (VAFSG), Nutrition education (NE), Nutrition education & Probiotic supplemented group (NE+PSG), Nutrition education & Value added food supplemented group (NE+VAFSG). No nutrition intervention was given to the pre-school children of corresponding control sub-groups.

The present study was carried out in three phases: Phase **I** (pre-intervention stage), Phase **II** (intervention stage) and Phase **III** (post-intervention stage). In Pre-intervention stage data regarding general information, anthropometry, biochemical, clinical, dietary habits, and nutrition knowledge was collected through the questionnaire developed specifically for the purpose. The enriched food preparations and nutrition education material for interventions were also developed. In second phase (intervention stage) children of experimental group were intervened with the various nutrition interventions for four months while no intervention was provided to corresponding control sub-groups children. In phase three (post-intervention stage) the impact of various nutrition interventions on nutritional status of the pre-school children was studied and statistically analysed (SPSS-version 18).

Prevalence of undernourishment among children before (zero day) imparting various nutritional trials was assessed. Age-wise prevalence data revealed that in the 3 years of age group 51.42 per cent and 41.66 per cent of the children were severely **under-weight** (malnourished) in experimental and control group respectively. Correspondingly, 40 and 41.66 per cent were moderately under-weight. For 4 years age group, maximum (89.74%) of the subjects in the experimental group and 100 per cent in the control group reported severely under-weight. All the children (100%) in 5 years and 6 years of age group were severely malnourished i.e. under-weight as per their age. As per **height-for-age** parameter, 37.14 percent and only 4.16 per cent of children of experimental and control group of 3 years of age group were severely stunted and 28.57 and 41.66 per cent of the pre-school children in experimental and control group were moderately stunted. Among 4 years of age group, maximum children of experimental group were severely stunted (79.48%) and 10.25 per cent of the experimental subjects belonged to moderate and normal category each, whereas in the control group all the children were severely stunted. Amongst 5 and 6 years age group children, majority (93.75% and 96.42%) of experimental and control preschool children were severely stunted while 6.25, 3.57 and 10 per cent of the respondents for all the groups except 6 years control group were moderately stunted. The data for **Weight-for-height** revealed that 22.85 per cent and 37.5 per cent of the children of the 3 years in the experimental and control respectively were severely wasted and similarly, 34.28 per cent (experimental) and 33.33 per cent (control) found to be moderately malnourished (wasted). For 4 years age group 17.94 and 41.17 per cent of the subjects were severely wasted in control and experimental group. Among 5 years age group, maximum children were moderate and severely malnourished in experimental (56.25%) and control group (46.42%), respectively. Correspondingly, in 6 years age-group equal per cent (40%) of the experimental subjects were moderately and severely malnourished (wasted) and only 20 per cent were falling in normal category. For control group maximum (48.38%) of pre-schoolers was moderately wasted and similar (25.80%) percentage of control subjects were in normal and severe category of undernutrition.

General information: As per age criteria, maximum (29.5%) children belonged to three years age group followed by four years (28%), five years (22%) and six years (20.5%). Almost equal percentages of male (49.5%) and female (50.5%) children participated in the study. Parental educational status showed that majority of the parents (68.5%) was illiterate. The fathers of the most of the respondents were working as labourers (58.5%), while mothers were not working (53%). Nearly two-third of the pre-school children (64%) belonged to nuclear family and one-third (36%) had joint family. Annual income data of the family showed that for majority (59.5%), family income was between Rs.70, 000-1, 00,000, one fourth had more than a lakh and rest (15.5%) were having between Rs. 50000-70000 income, annually. Maximum (97%) of the respondents were vegetarian and only 3 per cent were non-vegetarian. Frequency of the meal intake responses revealed that most of the pre-school children (42%) had two meals a day followed by once a day (30%) and only 28 per cent used to have three meals a day. Regarding skipping or missing the meal, responses were 77.5 per cent affirmative and that too usually. The most skipped meal was breakfast (39.35%) followed by lunch (38.06%) and evening meal (22.58%). The reasons for skipping the meal were attributed as not tasty (19.35%), monotonous (14.19 %), no appetite (43.22%), and lack of time (23.22%). Almost all the respondents (99.5%) nibbled; maximum between lunch and dinner (65.82%), some in between breakfast (19.59%), also in bedtime (14.57%) if available. As far as snacks were concerned, almost 100 per cent loved snacking and street food and most preferred were chips (31.5 %) followed by biscuits (28%), chocolates (21%) and crax (19.5%). Most liked street foods preference wise was chat/*tikki* (25%), *samosa /bread pakora* (23%), hotdogs/ burgers (21.5%), *golgappa* (19%) and *bhelpuri* (11%).

Clinical examination data revealed the presence of lack of lustre in hair (52%), pale conjunctiva in eyes (40%), normal lips (86%), and raw tongue (80.5%). Surprisingly most of the children had normal gums (88.5%), normal skin (87%) and normal nails (93%).

Summarization of **food intake data** revealed that cereal wheat was being consumed on routine basis, rice on alternate days and pulses on weekly basis. Bengal gram (53%) and red gram (44%) were the most preferred pulse followed by black gram, green gram and *rajma*. *Bathua*, spinach, fenugreek, potato, brinjal and tomato were

155

the most preferred vegetables by the respondents. None of the subjects were consuming fruits on the daily basis. Guava was most liked fruit being consumed by nearly one-half (46%) of the subjects on alternate days, whereas banana, mango, papaya and *jamun* were consumed more either weekly or monthly depending on availability (as reported). More than half (52%) of the pre-school children consumed cow's milk on daily basis and almost equal per cent of the children consumed milk alternately, weekly and monthly each and only 3.5 per cent were not in habit of consuming milk. Vanaspati and mustard oil were consumed on daily basis by 45 per cent and 31 per cent respectively, while butter (89.5%) and *desi* ghee (95.5%) was not consumed by the majority. All the respondents had sugar intake on daily basis, whereas maximum (46.5%) of the respondents did not consume jaggery.

Enriched food preparations like *Dalia, Poshtikbhel* and Biscuits were developed with different variations. 9-point hedonic scale was used for adjudging the best acceptable level of incorporation. The acceptable level of supplementation varied in all the food preparations, however mean sensory scores for all the characteristics declined on further supplementation beyond the accepted supplemented level. *Dalia* was best acceptable at 1.7 per cent spirulina supplementation, while acceptable level of *Poshtik bhel* was at 16.6 per cent with an incorporation of roasted soybean and biscuits were found to be most acceptable at 25 per cent supplementation with soybean flour.

The **daily food intake** of pre-school children was analysed before and after experimental period separately for 3 years and 4-6 years age groups. The result showed that the per cent intake of all the food groups except pulses and sugar by the children of control as well as experimental group was inadequate as compared to RDA before and after trial period. The mean per cent change of food intake among the experimental subjects of 3 years of age group was noticed maximum in milk and milk products (15.28%) followed by pulses (10.86%) and cereals (8.8%). No improvement was noticed in the control group among 3 years pre-school children after the completion of experimental trial. Maximum mean per cent change was found to be highest (10.16%) in other vegetables among food group. Whereas cereals, pulses, green leafy vegetables and fruits showed less improvement in 4-6 years in the experimental group. In comparison no improvement was reported in control group subjects.

Daily **nutrient intake** of pre-school children was found to be inadequate (except protein and iron in 3 years age group) as to RDA in experimental as well as control group. Further findings showed that improvement in mean per cent after the intervention trial was observed maximum for iron (15.02%) followed by protein (13.5%) and calcium (7.16%) in the experimental group while respective control group subjects reported further decreased per cent intake for all the nutrients except beta-carotene (10.14%) and calcium (1.1%). Pre-school children of 4-6 years age group reported highest increment for iron (15.3%) protein (13.2%) and beta-carotene (10.07%) after the 120 days of trial. A positive change or improvement was also perceived in the energy (3.2%), fat (5.77%) and calcium intake (7.37%). Further decreased in mean per cent change for all the respective nutrient was observed among corresponding control group subjects.

Anthropometric measurements

Height: On probiotic supplementation per cent change in height was three times more as compared to corresponding control sub-group. Growth in height was statistically significant ($p \leq 0.01$) after 2 and 4 months of probiotic feeding.

Experimental sub-groups subjects of VAFSG reported significant ($p \leq 0.01$) improvement for D/A and B/A. Control sub-groups of nutrition education and NE+PSG represented more per cent change in height as compared to corresponding experimental sub-groups with statically Significant ($p \leq 0.05$, $p \leq 0.01$) improvement. In VAFSG experimental group statistically significant ($p \leq 0.01$) growth of 0.2, 0.9 and 1.1 per cent was noticed after 0-60days, 60-120 and after 120 days respectively.

Perusal of the data for the control sub-groups of VAFSG, NE and NE+PSG suggested that during the whole study period, mean changes at different stages (B/D, D/A, and B/A) were not so representative, hence may be taken as natural growth which were however, statistically significant ($p \leq 0.01$, $p \leq 0.05$). Along with this, intervention with probiotics (PSG), value added foods (VAFSG) and nutrition education along with value added foods (NE+VAFSG) have also shown comparatively good sign of significant change ($p \leq 0.01$) in the mid and end of the study period.

Weight:

On NE+VAFSG supplementation highly significant (p≤0.01) improvement in weight was observed for B/D, D/A and B/A stages among experimental sub-group subjects as compared to non-significant change in weight for control sub-group subjects. Value-added food supplemented sub-group subjects showed significant (p≤0.01) improvement of 10.7, 7 and 18.5 per cent at 0, 60 and 120 days respectively. While control subgroup also showed weight gain of 4.8 and 4.4 per cent respectively B/D and B/A stages with significant impact. Nutrition education intervention group represented significant weight gain at all stages of trial period as compared to significant effect only at initial stage for control sub-group subjects. NE+PSG supplementation revealed significant (p≤0.01) weight gain of 13.6 per cent as compared to only 1 per cent for control sub-group. NE+VAFSG supplementation reported significant mean weight gain of 10.4,7 and 18.1 per cent at initial, mid and completion of intervention trial respectively as compared to negligible change reported among control sub-group at all the stages.

Further data analysis suggested almost same pattern of per cent weight gain for VAFSG and NE+VAFSG supplemented group followed by NE+PSG (13.6%) and PSG (12.8%). Significant improvement in weight was noticed among the experimental sub-groups of PSG, VAFSG, NE, NE+VAFSG at all stages of trial. However, control sub-group of VAFSG (B/D and B/A) and NE (B/D) also showed significant impact which can be explained as natural growth gain process.

BMI: Statistically significant (p≤0.01) improvement in body mass index parameters symbolised impact of various nutrition interventions VIZ. PSG, VAFSG, NE, NE+PSG and NE+VAFSG in all the experimental sub-groups. In control group significant change was noticed in VAFSG and NE+PSG at B/D and B/A stage whereas, NE showed significant change only at B/D stage.

Further analysis of the data confirmed VAFSG as the most impactful intervention with 17.2 per cent improvement followed by NE+VAFSG (16.7%), NE+PSG (13.2%), PSG (11.9%) and NE (7.7%). Hence, VAFSG was inferred as most effective intervention treatment.

Head circumference of the children showed almost negligible mean per cent change during all the stages of experimental trial. Statistical analysis indicated significant (p≤0.05) change only at D/A and B/A stage of PSG experimental group.

Chest circumference: The observed values of all the groups and sub-groups showed non-significant change except PSG experimental subjects (p≤0.01) at B/A and control sub-group of NE+VAFSG found significant (p≤0.05) change at D/A and B/A.

Arm circumference: Maximum gain in mean per cent was noticed among the experiment sub-groups of PSG (11.7%) followed by NE+PSG (5.8%) and VAFSG (4.3%) after (B/A) 120 days of experimental trial. Significant change was noticed in all the experimental trial groups except experimental sub-group of NE and control group of NE+VAFSG after completion of the trial.

Subscapular skin fold thickness Maximum (7.8%) mean per cent change was found only in VAFSG at B/A stage. The data generated through Statistical analyses found that significant (p≤0.01) increment in VAFSG and NE+VAFSG experimental group at D/A and B/A stage of nutrition intervention.

Triceps skin fold thickness: observed values revealed that the mean per cent change was gradually improved in all the experimental groups (except NE+PSG).Maximum mean per cent (7.2%) was observed in NE+VAFSG experimental group followed by PSG (7.2%), NE (4.2%) and VAFSG (4.1%) after 120 days of experimental trial. Whereas statistical analysis revealed that experimental group of PSG (D/A and B/A), VAFSG (B/D, D/A and B/A) and NE+VAFSG (D/A) were significantly (p≤0.01) improved.

TOTAL PROTEIN

PSG: The mean total protein values for subgroups (experimental and control) of probiotic supplemented group was 6.33±0.41g/dl,6.35±0.45g/dl, 6.51±0.42g/d and 6.04±0.81g/dl,5.99±0.82, 6.16±0.75g/dl before (0days), during (60 days) and after studied period (120days), respectively. In experimental sub-group gradual increase in total protein was observed during the whole duration of studied period, whereas in control sub-group maximum improvement was noticed at 60 days (during the study). The analysis further expressed non-significant change among both the sub-groups.

VAFSG: For value added food supplemented experimental sub-group, the mean values of total protein at zero day, 60 days and 120 days were 6.22±0.51g/dl, 6.37±0.31g/dl and 6.51±0.27g/dl, respectively. An increase in mean percentage as 2.5,

2.2 and 4.7 per cent was noticed as compared to almost nil improvement among control sub-group. Highly significant ($p \leq 0.01$) increment at all the three phases of the experimental trial confirmed good impact of VAFSG on the total protein content as per analysis.

NE: Nutrition education experimental sub groups presented very little (0.7%) non-significant improvement in total protein.

NE+PSG: The mean values for experimental group were 6.10 ± 0.37g/dl, 6.33 ± 0.45g/dl and 6.35 ± 0.48g/dl before (0day), during (60days) and after (120days) experimental trial, respectively. Experimental sub-group showed significant changes ($p \leq 0.01$) B/D (0-60days) and B/A (0-120days) the experimentation. While corresponding control group showed almost nil mean per cent change.

NE+VAFSG: The mean respective total protein values for the experimental sub-group were 6.03 ± 0.43g/dl, 6.10 ± 0.35g/dl and 6.35 ± 0.30g/dl before (0day), during (60days) and after 120 days of experimental trial. A steady increment in mean percentage of 1.2, 4.1 and 5.4 which was statistically highly significant ($p \leq 0.01$) reported during the different phases of trial among experimental sub-group.

Comparatively, mean per cent change was found to be highest among NE+VAFSG (5.4%), followed by VAFSG (4.7%), N.E + PSG (4.1%) and PSG (2.8%). Perusal of data further concluded that NE+VAFSG and VAFSG experimental sub-groups represented significant ($p \leq 0.01$) difference for B/D, D/A and B/A. For NE+PSG experimental group B/D and B/A have shown a good impact ($p \leq 0.01$). It is interesting to note that NE did not show any impact on total protein.

Serum Albumin

PSG: In the experimental sub-group the mean values were 3.79 ± 0.45g/dl, 3.79 ± 0.50g/dl, and 3.81 ± 0.49g/dl before (0day), during (60days), and after studied period (120days), respectively. The average serum albumin of control sub-group were 3.41 ± 0.64g/dl, 3.31 ± 0.70g/dl, and 3.43 ± 0.59g/dl before, during, and after the study, respectively. The effect of Probiotic supplementation was almost non existence in experimental group as evident in the analysis. Among corresponding control group improved mean percentage of 2.9 and 3.6 per cent was noticed which further reduced to only 0.6 per cent at the end of study which could be due to some sample error or other natural factors.

VAFSG: The observed mean values in the experimental group for before (0day), during (60days) and after (120days) were 3.64±0.60g/dl, 3.81±0.54g/dl and 3.89±0.52g/dl respectively. For control group there seems to be no changes up to the completion to the study. Feeding intervention sub-group showed significantly (p≤0.01) improved mean change of 6.9per cent for B/A (0-120days), 4.8 per cent for B/D (0-60days) and 2 per cent for D/A (60-120days).

NE: As per analysis controls as well as experimental group both did not show any impact of nutrition education on serum albumin.

NE+PSG: NE+PSG intervention has shown good impact in the experimental sub-group subjects, as evident by the mean values i.e. 3.38±0.35g/dl, 3.55±0.36g/dl and 3.83±0.28g/dl before (0day), during (60days) and after (120days), respectively. Whereas no change was found in control sub-group subjects. Further analysis showed mean per cent change of 13.3 (B/A), 7.9 (D/A) and 5.0 (B/D) in the experimental subjects which was highest amongst all the other intervention sub-groups. Furthermore, statistically significant (p≤0.01) values proved efficacy of combined nutrition education and probiotic supplementation.

NE+VAFSG: Among control sub-group respondents, almost negligible change in mean serum albumin values was observed during the different stages of intervention, the mean serum albumin values of experimental sub-group of NE+VAFSG were 3.29±0.47g/dl, 3.49±0.45g/dl and 3.69±0.51g/dl. A good percentage change of 12.3 per cent (B/A), 6.1 per cent (B/D) and 5.9 per cent in D/A of experimental sub-group represented significant (p≤0.01) effect as tested statistically.

The highest mean change was observed for B/A (13.3%) in N.E +PSG treatment group in the experimental sample followed by 12.3 per cent in B/A for experimental sample of N.E +VAFSG and 6.9 per cent in B/A of VAFSG experimental subjects. Most of the t values for serum albumin effect in rest of sub-groups were non-significant. It indicates that for both control as well as experimental sub-groups mean scores are showing some variations and may be attributed to sampling fluctuations as the groups are little bit at variant due to age, gender, height and weight etc, and may not affect the conduct of experiment. As a sum-up of the experiment it could be further pointed out that VAFSG, NE+PSG, and NE+VAFSG are standing in a same row. In other words, all these nutrition interventions can be thought to be equally affected on the experiment as per analysis. The study indicated that pattern of response is almost the same as that of total protein except that D/A was also showing a good impact of NE +PSG in experimental subgroups. The study indicated that NE + PSG has shown maximum efficacy of nutrition intervention in the estimation of serum albumin on the sample in the study area. For paired t-values VAFSG, NE+ VAFSG are showing similar trend for respective intervention on the serum albumin content in the blood sample in the study area.

Serum Globulin:

PSG: The mean serum globulin values of the experimental and control sub-groups were 2.54±0.64g/dl, 2.56±0.69g/dl, 2.70±0.64g/dl and 2.63±0.78g/dl, 2.68±0.89g/dl,2.73±0.66g/dl at 0 days, 60 days and 120 days, respectively. Gradual improvement in mean serum globulin values was noticed in both the sub-groups but comparatively, much more was reported in experimental sub-group with 6.3 per cent improvement at the end of the study period. Probiotic supplemented group showed maximum improvement of 6.3 per cent at the end of the study (120 days) but the improvement was non- significant statistically.

VAFSG: The observed mean values in the experimental sub-group were 2.58±0.59g/dl, 2.56±0.59g/dl, and 2.63±0.50g/dl during different stages of intervention and almost similar trend (3.03±0.37g/dl, 3.03±0.37g/dl, 3.02±0.36g/dl) was found in control sub-group. No significant impact was seen in studied period as mean percentage changes in control sub-group was almost of zero order and a change of 2.5 per cent for B/D (0-60days) in the experimental sub-group was noticed.

NE: The mean serum globulin values in the experimental sub-group were 3.14±0.52g/dl, 3.13±0.58g/dl and 3.16±0.94g/dl at before, during, and after nutrition education intervention, respectively. The observed respective mean values of the control group were 2.87±0.24g/dl, 2.88±0.23g/dl, and 2.89±0.25g/dl. The mean percentage change was negligible (0.8 and 0.5) in both the respective sub-groups hence; no significant increment was reported in the nutrition education intervention trial. Further analysis of the data revealed that the impact of nutrition education intervention was of the same pattern as that of PSG and VAFSG and cannot be taken as significant effect on mean serum globulin levels in the study area.

NE+PSG: The mean values of serum globulin in the experimental and control sub-groups were 2.73±0.49g/dl, 2.79±0.58g/dl,2.53±0.52g/dl and 2.80±0.42g/dl, 2.80±0.40g/dl, 2.80±0.40g/dl at starting, mid and completion of the intervention trial period, respectively. In control sub-group, there was effect of almost zero-order however in the experimental sub-group a mean per cent change of 9.3 per cent was observed for D/A (60-120days) and 7.3 per cent for B/A (0-120days) and these two are significantly different at 1 per cent and 5 per cent, respectively. Thus, NE+PSG intervention trial was effective significantly (p≤0.01) in improving the serum globulin level during the experimentation at the stages of D/A and B/A but not at B/D.

NE+VAFSG: Mean serum globulin value of the experimental sub-group as 2.74±0.64g/dl, 2.62±0.59g/dl, and 2.66±0.65g/dl at different stages of intervention trial. The respective average values of the control sub-group were 3.19±0.55g/dl,3.17±0.53g/dl, and 3.18±0.53. The control sub-group reported no specific trend, however experimental sub-group have shown a percentage change of 4.6 at the starting (B/D) with t value significant at 1 per cent.

The comparative analysis in indicated maximum mean per cent change of (9.3%) in case of experimental sub-group intervened with nutrition education along with probiotic supplementation. The perusal of the data further indicated that according to paired t test applied the t static significant improvement (p≤0.01), for D/A and B/A in experimental sample of NE +PSG and only B/D in experimental sample of NE +VAFSG (p≤0.01) were showing significant impact of nutrition interventions on serum globulin levels of respective subjects.

Haemoglobin:

PSG: The respective mean haemoglobin values in the probiotic supplemented experimental and control sub-groups were 8.71±1.12g, 8.86±1.13g, 9.67±1.06g and 8.56±1.58g, 8.60±1.44g, 8.76±1.41g at 0 days, 60 days and 120 days of the intervention trial period. In control sub-group, 2.3 per cent change was noticed in respect of haemoglobin parameter. However, a mean per cent change of 9.1per cent and 11.1 per cent, respectively for during and after were observed and corresponding t static was found to be significant (p≤0.01) increased for both (D/A and B/A) in the experimental trial. It indicates that the PSG is contributing towards improvement in haemoglobin level after 0-60 and 0-120 days of supplementation.

VAFSG: The average haemoglobin values of the in the experimental sub-group respondents showed an increased mean during (60days) and after the nutrition intervention i.e. from 8.84±1.85g to 9.35±1.68g and 10.42±1.52g. Control sub-group subject's mean haemoglobin values of 8.14±1.05g, 8.31±0.97g, and 7.97±1.06g depicted significant per cent change of 4.1 during D/A with t static of 2.80 (p≤0.01). Among experimental sub-group subjects, percentage mean of 17.9 per cent, 11.5 per cent and 5.8 per cent at 0-120 days (B/A), 60-120days (D/A) and 0-60days (B/D), respectively showed statistically significant (p≤0.01) improvements. Further analysis confirmed the contribution of value added food supplementation trial as a quiet effective in enhancing mean haemoglobin per cent level during all the three stages in the studied sample. The result indicated that there was a significant (p≤0.01) increment in haemoglobin indicator of the respondents after feeding them with different types of supplemented mixture.

NE: The respective mean haemoglobin values of the experimental and control sub-groups were 8.66±1.45g, 8.93±1.28g, 9.45±1.05 and 8.66±0.92g, 8.65±0.74g, 8.53±0.75g at zero day, 60days and 120 days of nutrition education intervention trial period. Control sub-group depicted no significant effect but for experimental group, statistically significant (p≤0.01) changes of 5.8 per cent and 9.1 per cent was observed (p≤0.01) respectively after 60 days and 120 days of trial period. Perusal of the data revealed some positive impact of nutrition education trial on haemoglobin level of the children which can be acknowledged.

NE+PSG: Among the experimental sub-group subjects improving average haemoglobin values i.e. from 8.80±1.27g to 10.33±1.01g, and 11.06±0.94g towards the completion of the trial period were observed. Significantly (p≤0.01) highly improved change in mean per cent i.e. 25.7 per cent (B/D) and 17.4 per cent (B/A) was noticed among children intervened with nutrition education and probiotic supplementation. On the contrary, negligible mean per cent change was observed for respective control group

NE+VAFSG: The observed haemoglobin mean values of the experimental sub-group (9.75±1.62g, 9.87±1.37g, 11.01±1.09g) represented improving trend during the experimentation period. Maximum mean per cent change of 11.6% and 13% in haemoglobin values obtained for two phases i.e. during (0-60 days) and after the supplementation trial were observed to be highly significant (p≤0.01). In the control sub-group as steady improvement was not noticed (8.36±1.03g, 8.39±0.89g, and 8.20±1.05g), hence no significant change at any stage of the study period was observed.

In the experimental sub-groups PSG- D/A and B/A (P≤0.01), VAFSG- B/D, D/A and B/A all (P≤0.01), N.E- D/A and B/A (P≤0.05), N.E +PSG all subgroups i.e. B/D, D/A and B/A (p≤0.01) found to be showing a good impact of nutrition interventions on the growth of haemoglobin level of the experimental sub samples. Whereas corresponding control sub-groups did not report any significant change except VAFSG that was only for D/A (60-120 days) of experimental trial.

The study has clearly indicated that nutrition interventions of almost all the experimental sub-groups have shown favourable results and can be taken as a good response of nutrition interventions in the study area.

Haemoglobin, one of the most important indicators has been observed to be affected by the nutritional interventions. It is suggested that the highest mean percentage change in haemoglobin of the order of 25.7 per cent was identified in the experimental sample of N.E+PSG. This indicates that this nutrition intervention has affected most in the experimental sample compared to all other interventions. Apart from this intervention sub-group, some others have also shown good impact i.e. 17.9 % by VAFSG, 13 % by N.E+ VAFSG and 11.1% by PSG. As it evident through highly significant values of t-static (p≤0.01) that NE+PSG and VAFSG have shown much greater impact as seen during the entire experiment period and could be regarded as real effects of nutrition interventions in the study area.

Nutrition Education: After imparting nutrition education to the experimental sub-group mean knowledge, attitude and practice (KAP) scores of the mothers showed significant increment (p≤0.01) with mean percentage of 340.62, 316.21 and 406.25 per cent respectively. On the contrary mean KAP scores of control sub-group reported respective negative per cent change of -36.36, -1.86 and -2.09.

NE+PSG: Mean KAP score before (0day) and after intervention trial (120 days) were 1.15±0.93, 11.05±0.88, 11.95±1.53 and 7.45±1.23, 17.40±1.39, 18.00±1.33 respectively. Mean percent change was maximum for knowledge scores (547.8%) followed by attitude (57.46%) and practice (50.6%) scores. Statically highly significant (p≤0.01) difference between before and after intervention trial scores indicated sufficient gain in knowledge, attitude and practice scores among the experimental group. Corresponding control sub-group subjects showed gain in knowledge scores (50%) only and that too was non-significant.

NE+VAFSG: The mean KAP scores were 1.45±0.99, 11.40±0.99, 11.55±1.09 and 6.95±1.57, 18.40±1.04, 17.85±1.22 respectively in the beginning (0day) and on completion (120 days) of intervention trial period. Gain of 379.3 per cent in knowledge scores, 61.4 per cent in attitude scores and 54.5per cent in practice scores showed highly significant (p≤0.01) improvement. Control sub-group subjects to whom no education was provided represented nil improvement in their respective scores.

KAP SCORES: All the mothers of control group scored very poor grades (0-5 marks) before and after experimental trial. Before imparting nutrition education majority of the mothers of respective experimental group (65%) scored very poor marks (0-5) and almost 1/3rd of the subjects scored marks in between 6-10 i.e. poor marks. After 120 days of nutrition education intervention increment in the scores was noticed i.e. 10 per cent of the mothers improved to excellent scores category (26-30), 3/4th scored very good marks (21-25) and 30 per cent of the subjects recorded good marks (16-20).

NE+PSG: Before commencing the nutrition intervention trial most of the mothers (3/4th) were categorized in very poor category i.e. 0-5 marks followed by poor category (1/4th subjects). After providing nutrition education for 120 days, one half of the mothers (50%) improved to very good category (21-25) followed by good category i.e. 16-20 marks (30%) and 1/5th of the mothers improved to excellent category which was nil before nutrition education intervention. On the contrary similar trend of marks was observed regarding KAP scores among control group subjects.

NE+VAFSG: In the beginning stage most of the subjects reported very poor (65%) and poor (35%) KAP scores which improved to good (15%), very good (65%) and excellent (20%) category on completion of four months of nutrition education intervention. All the mothers of the control group remained in very poor category (0-5 marks).Comparatively maximum improvement in KAP scores was found among NE+VAFSG followed by NE+PSG and NE

The result of assessment of nutritional status before and after imparting nutrition interventions revealed that **Weight-for-age** among 3years age-group 51.42 per cent and 41.66 per cent of the pre-school children were severely underweight in experimental and control group respectively, before commencing the nutrition intervention trialsIn experimental group of 4 years age group maximum (89.74%) of the experimental subjects was severely underweight. All the respondents (100%) of experimental and control group for 5 and 6 years of age group falling in the category of severely underweight. For height-for-age the result revealed that pre-school children of experimental and control group of 3 years of age group 37.14 per cent and 4.16 per cent were severely stunted. However in the experimental group of 4 years of age group maximum (79.48%) pre-schoolers were severely stunted. Almost all the respondents of 5 and 6 years of the age group were severely stunted. The data for Weight-for-height revealed that 22.85 per cent and 37.5 per cent of the subjects of the 3 years age group in the experimental and control were severely malnourished (wasted) and at the same time 34.28 per cent in experimental and 33.33 per cent in control group found to be moderately malnourished. After supplementation none of the experimental subjects were severely underweight in 3 years age group. Comparatively less improvement was observed among control group of all the age-groups. In 5 and 6 years age-group $3/8^{th}$ (37.5%) and $3/10^{th}$ (30%) per cent decline was noticed in the experimental subjects of severe underweight category. Results for height-for-age revealed that negligible change for all the control subjects of 3-6 years age group. While experimental subjects showed some impact of supplementation in improving the nutrition status. Subsequently efficacy of intervention was observed in sample units of experimental group for weight-for-height showed maximum increment 60 per cent among 6 years subjects followed by 50, 48.85, 38.16 per cent in 5, 4 and 3 years respectively.

The overall prevalence of underrnutrition after imparting nutrition interventions revealed that maximum (47%) per cent was declined from severity form of undernutrition whereas 25 and 22 per cent increment was observed in moderate and normal category. The percentage for height-for-age revealed that 16, 16 and 68 per cent of the respondents were in the category of normal, severely and moderately malnourished before imparting nutrition interventions, whereas increment (2% and 7%) was found in normal and moderate category after the experimental trial completed. The data for weight-for-height revealed that in the experimental group 46 per cent increment was observed in the normal category of weight-for-height. Only 8 and 5 per cent of the respondents were in moderate and severe category after 120 days of experimental trial.

ASSESSMENT OF NUTRITIONAL STATUS OF CHILDREN (3-6 YEARS) OF DISTRICT KARNAL AND DISTRICTKURUKSHETRA

General Information

Name of respondent: …………...

Date of Birth: ....

Class: …………………………………………………..………

Sex: Male/ Female……………………………………………….

☐Parental Education:

    A) Illiterate

    B) Primary Education

    C) Matric

    D) Intermediate

    E) Graduate

☐Father Occupation:

    A) Businessman

    B) Serviceman

    C) Labor

☐Mother Occupation:

    A) Working

    B) Not- Working

☐Family Type:

    A) Joint

    B) Nuclear

    C) Extended

☐Income:

    A) 50,000-70,000

    B) 70,000-1,00,000

    C) More than lakh

☐House Type

    A) Katcha

    B) Pucca

    C) Jugghi

Dietary Habits

1. Eating Habit

    a) Vegetarian

    b) Non- Vegetarian

    c) Eggetarian

2. If non- Vegetarian which Non- Veg. do you consume?

    a) Chicken b) Mutton c) fish d) pork

3. Frequency of consuming non-veg

    a) Daily b) Once a week c) Twice a week d) Once in a month

4. If eggetarian frequency of consuming egg

    a) Daily b) once a week c) twice a week d) once in a month

5. Number of meals you consume in a day

a) One b) Two c) Three

9. Do you skip meal?

    (a) Yes (b) no

10. If yes then

    (a) Daily (b) Usually (c) Sometimes

11. Which meal do you skip most?

    (a) Breakfast (b) lunch (c) dinner

12. Reason of skipping meal

    (a) Not tasty (b) monotonous (c) lack of time (d) Not feeling hungry

13. Do you nibble?

      (a) Yes (b) No

14. If yes then what time?

      (a) In between breakfast and lunch (b) in between lunch and dinner

      (c) In between dinner and bed time

15. Do you like snacking?

      (a) Yes (b) no

16. What do you prefer in snacking?

17. Do you like junk food?

      (a)Yes (b) no

18. If yes then what do you like in junk/street food?

A) Anthropometric Measurements:

Height (in cm)………   BMI…………

Weight (in kg)………   Arm Circumference (cm)…………

Head circumference (cm)………   Chest circumference (cm)…………….

Triceps skinfold thickness (mm)…………. MUAC (cm)………………

Subscapular skinfold thickness (mm)……….

B) Clinical assessment:

Organs	Deficiency signs	No. of Subjects	Percentage
Hair	Lack of lustre		
	Dyspigmentation		
	Normal Hair		
Eyes	Pale Conjunctiva		
	Bitot's Spot		
	Night Blindness		
	Normal eyes		

Lips	Angular Scars
	Normal pink lips
Tongue	Scarlet
	Raw tongue
	Normal tongue
Teeth	Mottled enamel
	Caries
	Normal teeth
Gums	Spongy gums
	Normal gums
Skin	Skin Xerosis
	Pale
	Normal skin
Nails	Brittle nails
	Ridged nails
	Normal nails

DIETARY INFORMATION:

Food intake frequency for the child

SR.NO.	FOOD STUFF	DAILY	ALTERNATELY	WEEKLY	MONTHLY

1. Cereals

Wheat

Rice

Maize

Bajra

Any other

2. Pulses

Bengal gram

Black gram

Green gram

Red gram

Moong

Rajma

Soyabean dal

3. Roots and Tubers

Potato

Carrot

Onion

Garlic

Ginger

Radish

Turnip

Any other

4. Other vegetables

Tomato

Brinjal

Beans

Cauliflower

Bitter gourd

Ridge gourd

Bottle gourd

Peas

5. Green Leafy Vegetables

Spinach

Fenugreek

Mint

Coriander

Brathua

Any other

6. Fruits

Guava

Banana

Orange

Mango

Papaya

Apple

Jammun

Any other

7. Milk and milk products

Buffalo's milk

Cow's milk

Curd

Cottage cheese

Butter milk

Butter

Any other

8. Fats and edible oil

Desi ghee

Vanaspati

Mustard Oil

 Any other (specify)

9. Sugar and jaggery

CONCLUSION

The three value-added products namely *Dalia*, biscuits and *Poshtik bhel* were developed and standardized using spirulina, soya flour, and roasted soyabean with an aim to improve nutritional level of undernourished children. The value-added products were organoleptically acceptable and liked very well by the pre-school children. The supplementation of the value-added products to the experimental subjects' over a period of 120 days reduced the percentage of severe form undernourishment to moderate and normal category.

Feeding of value-added products to the subjects for 120 days resulted into positive responses in anthropometric (height, weight, BMI, arm circumference) and bio-chemical parameters (total protein, serum albumin, serum globulin and haemoglobin) in all the experimental subjects. Out of five experimental sub-groups, the groups intervened with VAFSG, NE+PSG and NE+VAFSG showed the highest positive response in all the bio-chemical parameters except serum globulin. Only NE+PSG experimental group showed impact on serum globulin level during (0-60 days) and after the nutrition intervention trial (120days). Maximum increase in serum albumin was noticed in NE+PSG followed by NE+VAFSG and VAFSG experimental subjects. Whereas maximum increase in haemoglobin was observed among the experimental subjects of NE+PSG followed by VAFSG, NE+VAFSG and PSG respectively. Comparison of the data further revealed that the feeding of probiotics along with nutrition education and value-added food and NE+VAFSG was more effectual in escalating the levels of haemoglobin and serum albumin. While results of anthropometric parameters concluded that PSG, VAFSG, NE+PSG and NE+VAFSG experimental subjects had effective gain of the weight. Perusal of the data facts further revealed that all the experimental trials (NE) are effectual in respect of BMI after 120 days of nutrition interventions.

At the end of the experiment after a period of 120 days, knowledge, attitude, and practice scores were assessed among 60 mothers in control and 60 in experimental group spread over three nutrition interventions given to children under experimental group as NE, NE+PSG, NE+VAFSG. It was noticed that all the three nutrition interventions have a good score to enhance knowledge, attitude and practice characteristics of the mothers of children under study. It is clear from the study that the attitude plays a negative role for NE in control group and a good effect in experimental groups for NE+PSG as well as NE+VAFSG also. This means that the mothers of the subjects gained a good knowledge after imparting nutrition education over the period of 120 days.

The KAP scores of nutrition education of experimental subject's mothers showed a highly significant increment after the experimental trial of four months. In addition to above, it was found that almost in all the control groups, most were in the very poor category of response (0-5). However, for NE, 3 per cent were scoring good (16-20) and 15 per cent very good and only 2 per cent were graded as excellent. Similarly for NE+PSG, 6 per cent were under the category of good and 4 per cent in excellent. In NE+VAFSG group, 3, 3, and 4 per cent were in good, very good, and excellent categories, respectively. The prevalence of undernutrition (underweight, stunting and wasting) among the preschool children intervened with various nutrition intervention trials decreased, whereas the percentage of severe, moderate undernutrition among control subjects remained unchanged.

Thus it indicates that supplementation of the value-added food products and imparting nutrition education to the mothers of the children is helpful to improve the nutritional status of the individuals. At the same time, supplemented value-added food products are not only beneficial to improve nutritional status but also fulfil the daily requirement of essential nutrients required for the body to remain healthy. Hence, value-added food products to children and nutrition education to the mothers of the children could be promoted in the community as one of the strategies of food based approach for improving nutritional status and eradicating undernutrition from the community.

CPSIA information can be obtained
at www.ICGtesting.com
Printed in the USA
BVHW051511180423
662564BV00014B/1034

9 781805 258216